Secrets
of a
Svelte and
Healthy Body

A guide for the young, the old, the healthy, the handicapped, the discouraged, and the broken.

Nina Kay

ISBN-13: 978-1503375543
ISBN-10: 1503375544

DEDICATION

This book is dedicated to everyone seeking heath and wellness. A svelte and healthy body is your birthright.

CONTENTS

ACKNOWLEDGMENTS

This book is written for the love of family, friends, and for everyone who struggles with health and weight management.

I would like to acknowledge everyone who offered me insights on health and wellness along the journey. Regarding official references, every effort has been made to reference the internet websites and other sources used for this book. If any reference is missing, it is an honest error or omission and not an error of commission.

The seeds for my journey into health were planted by father. He instilled a love of knowledge and understanding within me and my siblings. My father was always reading and trying to understand life, health, religion, history, mathematics, computers, physics, the universe etc. This was the reasons I kept searching for the answers to my health concerns. It took much longer for me to figure out all the pieces of the puzzle. Having done so, I share my experience and knowledge with my readers.

This book is for all individuals who are seeking health and fitness. Some are not finding easy answers to their problems. There are others who are suffering from debilitating or life threatening illnesses. The greatest hope is that the secrets presented in this book offers some insights for everyone.

1 INTRODUCTION

In the end, health is true wealth

We are all a product of what we eat, how we live, and how we chose to spend our free time. Indeed, we are also a product of our genes, our upbringing, our socio-economic environment, our home and work environment, and a multitude of other factors. Among these, it is what we consume, how we live, how we think, and who we surround ourselves with that can be adapted and positively impact our daily lives.

In order to achieve health, a careful review of what we eat and how we live is required. In this context, it is important to:

- Establish a lifestyle that helps build and maintain a svelte and healthy body. In addition, it is important to maintain a connection with nature each day, even if it is for a few minutes or hours.
- Review and reorganize priorities so that they reflect what we want out of life.
- Surround ourselves with caring and

supportive individuals.

- Find satisfaction in each day, even if it is because of gazing at a flower, listening to a nice song, hearing a joke, engaging in a good conversation, reading a noteworthy article, or watching a movie brings about a good feeling.

Life is simply too short not to do so and it is most abundant when following a path that helps us live healthy and fruitful lives and allows us to thrive (and not just survive) each day.

The primary focus of this book is to to uncover the secrets of a lifestyle that helps build and maintain a svelte and health body. Some mention is made of the other guidelines but the primary aim is helping everyone achieve a svelte and healthy body.

Though it may not seem possible to some, it is a for all humans, despite their genetic makeup, family upbringing, socio economic status, etc. to achieve excellent health. The purpose of this book to help you achieve this birthright.

Do not go on another diet without reading this book— Not the vegetarian, the paleolithic, the fruitarian, the vegetarian, the vegan nor any other diet!

2 MY STORY

We humans are like fruits, trees, plants, flowers
We are like all other living things
We are born and ripen to a peak
Slowly we start to shrivel and finally return to our source.
We are part and parcel of the continuous cycle of life
But, amazingly we also dream, imagine, and seek knowledge and
understanding of life and the universe
These are among the things that make us special

I suffered from lack of energy my entire life until I found the way to build a healthy and svelte body. As a child, a teenager and as an adult, I never felt healthy until I experimented on my own body and learned the secrets of health and wellness. These secrets represent years and years of searching and experimenting with different ways to achieve health and wellness.

Most of my life, I barely had enough energy to get through the day. At specific points in my life, and on occasion, I would feel good and energized. Most of the time, however, I felt tired, anxious and lacking in sufficient energy. These feelings led me to a very long journey—

lasting more than 35 years—trying to figure out how to attain health and vigor.

I recall being called fat at a very young age. When I was about 5 or 6 years old, some older male relatives used to tease me about my big stomach. They also teased me about many other things. My parents never said anything to me or them (I am not sure if my parents were aware of these comments but they affected me deeply). These relatives also subjected me to sexual abuse, which tarred my self image well into my mid-40s, when I was finally able to put these horrible memories behind me.

I remember having a big round stomach as a young child and being teased and really hating it. As I got a bit older and was busy with school and family responsibilities, I managed my weight much better. I was not emotionally strong but was able to maintain my weight a bit better. I was slowly building some level of emotional strength as well. By this time, the relatives who used to tease me were not around anymore. However, I was still quite young and unprepared for how I would feel as the years progressed.

During my teen years, I was very busy with school. I also held a full time job and helped raise younger siblings. In addition, I was involved in a host of family responsibilities. By age 16, I was very busy but felt a little better as I was more in charge of what I ate than in the past. This was good as I was able to "grow up" on my own and gain some level of control. I remember eating a lot of cabbage and pimento cheese. I worked in a restaurant after school and these foods were among the foods readily available to me that I chose to eat. Unfortunately, I also drank a lot of diet soda on a regular basis, which was the new fad at the time. My parents did not bring diet drinks into the house. However, I had free access to soda and fountain drinks at the restaurant where I worked. I drank diet soda as it was marketed as the answer to being slim. Though I was not fat as a teenager, I did not think I had a good figure. I also did not feel sufficiently healthy. I carefully watched what I ate, but I never felt strong or energetic.

Peer pressure as well as long work hours kept me slim. Despite having a good figure, I did not feel as good as I should have at that age. I wondered if it was stress or something more that kept me from feeling my best. Being a teen can be stressful, particularly when it come to body image and self esteem. There were also a number of other overwhelming family stresses during my childhood that impacted my self image negatively.[1] I often felt anxious and lacked a sense of well-being. I also did something that a lot of teenagers were doing—I occasionally consumed laxatives so that I would not gain weight. Perhaps this is why I was not a fat teenager and yet felt miserable even though I did not look it. My body was starving due to lack of proper nutrition.

A teenager can hide a lot of things that they are doing and they do not necessarily understand the consequences of abusing their body. (I grew up before the age of the internet and thus access to information was very sparse, but even today's teenagers and adults do not always get the correct information through the internet.) There is too much marketing and special interest that govern the information provided to the general public. But, thankful there are a few websites that reveal the truth.

As a teenager, I recall one high school classmate getting thiner and thiner each day. At the time I did not know what was happening to her, but she did not look right and there seemed to be a serious problem. I did not understand her situation at that point in my life and the internet was not in existence. I am not sure if her parents, teachers or others close to her understood the problem. In hindsight I know that she was suffering from anorexia nervosa. She was extremely gaunt and sickly and needed help. It was also a time when anorexia was not widely

---

[1] Though I had repressed my memories at the time, I was sexually abused as a young child, which impacted me throughout my life.

known. I hope and pray that someone got her some help before it was to late.

After finishing high school, I left home to attend university. Life there was incredibly busy and even more stressful. I was extremely unprepared for the external world into which I was thrust as I was raised in a very sheltered home. I also lacked sufficient financial resources and had to work most days in order to have money for food, rent, books, etc.

I had a busy class and study schedule, coupled with a rigorous work schedule. At the same time, family problems were escalating at home and I could not understand what was happening to me, my life, and my family. Being far away from home, my thoughts often drifted and I would worry a lot and felt stressed out on a daily basis. I did find some ways to target stress in order to maintain my focus on school. When I was not studying, eating or sleeping, I was generally working. However, I found time to go for 2 to 3 mile jogs a few times a week to help alleviate anxiety and stress. Fun and rest were reserved for Saturday nights. In the end, I was generally bored on Saturday nights as I did not have a personal life. I can safely say that I did not have a social life in college—I was unprepared to have one emotionally, financially, practically, and physically.

There were many good looking, well-dressed women at university. Comparatively, I was average in size and did not have the money to dress like my peers. I wanted to be more like them and my one any only way was to diet so that I could look good. I tried various and sundry diets advertised in magazines that I perused in the library. Clearly, I did not feel good about myself and my body and I did not feel healthy. Occasionally, I used to spend my very limited and hard earned money buying mail order diets pills and elixirs that did not do much for my figure and only made my heart race faster and my meager pocket book lighter. The mail order remedies did not help in anyway. They were just a waste of money. I often felt enormous stress and anxiety, which were only exasperated by my experimental diets as most of the diet pills increased my heart rate and thus anxiety.

I do not recall ever being comfortable in my skin during my undergraduate years. I was very unsure of myself and would anticipate that many people looked at me in this manner. I did not have the experience to be in the world and I certainly did not have the money nor the time. My body image was extremely poor. Looking back, I also had some food sensitivities back then but did not know what they were. I also had some health issues that did not get resolved for many years as my parents never took me to a doctor when I was young. I suffered from extreme stress and I had a difficult relationship with food, life, and the external world in general.

Unfortunately, many women in college had a complex relationship with food. I recall one dorm mate eating 3 or 4 boxes of Mint Milano cookies in one sitting with the sole intention of developing an aversion for such cookies. She loved Mint Milano cookies and wanted to "sicken" her taste buds so that she would no longer eat them. I hope that she was successful in killing her taste for these cookies. Also, during exam time, many women turned to smoking and overeating to manage anxiety and stress. To alleviate my anxiety, I would binge eat and later feel horrible. I would chew crackers and then spit them out. (At least, I was no longer doing laxatives.) I did not have much money so it was easy to buy unhealthy food as it was generally cheaper and seemed to be more filling. Nevertheless, despite lacking money, I binged on food that cost me money. Why? Because I was anxious, alone, stressed, depressed and not comfortable with my body, my life, and myself.

Graduate school seemed a bit easier, but still very challenging and stressful. The stress level was somewhat higher than my undergraduate years, but by that time I had learned to manage stress somewhat better. Nevertheless, I was not particularly fit nor healthy. I spent most of my time in class or at work and thus was always on the go. I recall several times working for 35 to 40 hours straight at the hospital intensive care unit in order to make enough money to pay for rent, books, food, etc. Perhaps I was lacking in sleep, which contributed to my general sense of poor health.

Upon entering the world of work after my graduate studies, it was imperative that I dress well. Thus, keeping a presentable figure in order to dress well became a primary goal. Also, as I was in debt with massive student loans, once I started buying business attire, it was important that I maintain my size so that I could wear my clothes for many years. I had an extremely limited budget to the point that I had to control how many times in a month I could afford to do laundry. I had to pay to do laundry at my apartment and thus I had to have funds to use the washer and dryer in the basement. Being able to fit into my clothes once I purchased them was also imperative. I worked very long hours and under an inordinate amount of stress. I tried to eat what I considered healthy at the time and to maintain a decent work, rest and sleep schedule. But, it was nearly impossible to do given the long work hours, the long daily commute, the travel requirements of the job, the uncertainty of client assignments, family commitments, etc. I also struggled to have a personal life, which was nearly impossible. I had to keep my focus on my career as I needed to pay off the extensive college loans I had accumulated. My family did not seem to have the money to pay for my loans and I needed to pay my debts. The above notwithstanding, I was still relatively young, and could get by on very little sleep and was able to maintain simple eating habits since I was generally eating alone. After a full day of work until 8 pm or so and then commuting home on the train and bus, I would settle down at about 10 pm. Often I would have a light dinner around 10 pm, comprising a plate of vegetables (or a warm bowl of oatmeal in the winter months), and then go to bed as I had to start the entire routine next day early morning. I did not feel particularly healthy and always felt stressed.

I kept this pace for nearly 27 years. I worked hard and faithfully, at the expense of my health and happiness. I mostly worked 6 days a week. Despite giving my life to my career, I lost my job at each company where I worked. I dedicated myself to the firm fully and each time I was pushed out of the firm for an extraneous reason. This was the cut throat and prejudiced world in which I worked. Each time I lost my job, my stress level shot up. Then, one day, all of a sudden, I lost my last job after working there for over 22 years. Upon filing a legal case against the firm, I found out that I lost my job as I had done too good a job. I could not believe it. How does one get fired at the peak of their career for doing a job well. I was given only a few weeks notice and lost half my pension as a result. Shortly thereafter, literally within a month or so, the 2008 financial crisis broke out and companies stopped hiring. I felt lost and my anxiety and stress went through the roof. I started to sit at home staring at the walls all day and feeling lost. I did not eat much, but I started to gain an inordinate amount of weight.

Soon, I was unable to bend to pick up stuff from the floor and my shoulders would ache all day and night. My teeth and gums started to hurt on all four sides of my mouth, I felt sharp and piercing stomach pains after eating solid food. Every time I ate grapes, apples or anything with tough skin or fiber, I would regurgitate these foods. While in the restroom, I often felt as if there was a sharp knife in my stomach and intestines, and I would have to lie on the bathroom floor in order to stretch my "insides" so that pain could subside. I almost fainted many times due to the pain. I made many changes to my die, which helped with the intestinal pains. But, even after making these dietary changes based on my physician and nutritionist's recommendations, I still did not feel fully well. Several times, I almost fainted while driving. This dangerous and I realized I had to do something. I also had extreme vertigo while baby sitting a nephew and niece and I had to drop to the floor in order to stop myself from falling. Often, while driving at night I could not see properly as I was losing night vision. I was also gaining weight at an extreme rate and could no longer get out of bed easily as my enlarged and "flowing" belly made it hard for me to easily get out of bed. My asthma continued to worsen as well. Climbing up and down the stairs was also challenging. I was barely turing 50, but suddenly I had the body, the teeth, and the eyes of a 75 year old. In short, my body had succumbed to extreme stress and dietary imbalance and my organ systems and senses were short circuiting. It was as if a lighting bolt had hit me.

I was miserable and felt I was losing myself. At this point I felt compelled to figure out what was wrong with me and what I could do to save myself. Within a year of starting to feel direly ill, I found out that I had: (1) non-alcoholic fatty liver disease, (2) celiac disease and thus could no longer tolerate gluten, (3) hypothyroidism, (4) colon polyps, which were removed via colonoscopy, and (5) severe asthma, which my allergist refused to treat as he could not understand the cause of my condition. Another allergist gave me allergy shots for over a year, but they did not help in the end. I was diagnosed with allergies to a multitude of trees, fruits, cats, dust and dander, etc. I was also highly deficient in several vitamins and minerals, including Vitamin B12 and Vitamin D. My liver enzymes were completely out of whack and my intestines were highly inflamed. These problems were overwhelming to deal with but I had to find solutions if I was going to survive.

I slowly started to follow the doctor's recommendations for celiac disease and took thyroid medication and I started to feel somewhat better. I thought that I had found the answers to my health problems and hoped that I would soon feel much better. It turns out that this was just one part of the answer, but not the full pathway to health—it was just the tip of the iceberg. Removing gluten and all sugary drinks from my diet altogether did help with the severe stomach pains and it also reduced some of the anxiety. However, I still had inflammation in my digestive system, and I had non-alcoholic fatty liver disease, which was getting worse with time. Thus, my stomach continued to be inflamed on a gluten free diet. Although, admittedly I did feel somewhat better and my teeth started to not hurt as much. In the meantime, I developed two additional conditions: pre diabetes and rheumatoid arthritis.

It took me an additional 8 years to figure it out. I researched and tried almost every diet as well as combination of diets, e.g., raw food diet, fruitarian diet, vegetarian diet, vegan diet, Atkins style high protein / ketosis diet. I tried a host of other remedies as well. I also spoke to friends and acquaintances who were trying various diets including the paleolithic and the Atkins diets about their experience with these diets. I went to doctors for many years to get my blood tests. I had follow up consultations due to fatty liver disease, pre-diabetes, etc. In the end, it was the persistent trial and error that ultimately led me to health and fitness. I ultimately lost more than 50 pounds, got rid of my pre diabetic condition, fatty liver disease and severe asthma, and improved my muscle strength, flexibility, and endurance. I finally started to feel better than I had in a long time.

It took too long, but at least I figured it out. Now I feel compelled to share my findings with my readers. I truly feel for anyone who is suffering from ill health or is overweight—I know what it feels like. I am here to share my story and hope that it will help others in someway.

In the chapters that follow, I explain the kind of diet that one needs to follow to build a svelte body and get healthy. I am not a doctor, so please consult your doctor as necessary. However, read this book carefully as the advice offered here will help anyone.

3 THE CLEANSE

The first step in regaining health is to clean the body and, in particular, the digestive tract. Whether it is illness, general weight management problems, or sheer curiosity, the protocol for building a healthy body is the same.

First and foremost, start by cleaning out you system with simple foods and water for at least three days. A body, like a plumbing system, is filled with debris which needs to be cleaned out periodically. Our bodies get clogged when we eat foods that are not ideal for us. All of us have consumed such foods in our life. We also don't know how our bodies are reacting to specific foods unless we clean out the digestive system. (It should noted that in some cases a more comprehensive elimination diet may be required whereby all foods are off limits and each food is introduced to the body one by one over a 3 to 5 day period to determine how the body reacts.) Allergy tests as well as other medical tests can also be provide some information on food and related allergies. Regardless, a cleanse is recommended in order to reset the body.

The digestive system needs to be "flushed out" to clean the digestive tract by running only basic foods through it.

This will ultimately allow the digestive system to run more efficiently and increase energy in the body. Flushing the digestive system is best done by consuming simple foods and fresh water. Certainly, if you wish to fast for a day or two that is fine, but it is not required. Your body heals best when it is properly nourished and managed with tender loving care. Indeed, occasional fasting is also fine and it can be quite helpful in giving the body and the digestive tract a rest and time to reset.

Some of the simplest foods to consume during the cleanse include bananas, apples, oranges, berries, tomatoes, lettuce, greens, cucumbers, celery, and nuts and seeds. There are many other simple foods that you may choose to consume for the three-day period. Drinks that are allowed during this short cleansing period include water, which may be taken cold, room temperature or warm. In addition, it is fine to flavor the water with lemon, lime, fresh mint or other herbs etc. Herbal tea is also acceptable.

It is, however, important to exclude foods that are processed. This means no bread, pasta, rice etc. Potatoes, meat, fish, eggs, and cheese should also be excluded. Coffee, tea (except herbal tea) chocolate, fruit juices etc are prohibited for the three day period. Smoothies are allowed if they are made with whole fruits and vegetables, i.e., the fiber is retained. Needless to say, alcohol is prohibited. The cleansing process only lasts a short while, but it will commence the reset process.

As far as liquids are concerned, it is important to hydrate your body. This means drinking adequate amounts of water. Proper hydration is important from now onwards as water is essential to life. Water is needed to aid the digestion process and it is needed to keep the skin supple.

In addition to following a strict eating and drinking regimen for three days, ensure that you get adequate sleep. A minimum of 8 hours of sleep is required. If needed, you may wish to sleep longer in order to give your body a full rest. The best time to fall asleep is a few hours after dark and get up shortly after the sun rises. Nevertheless, follow a sleep schedule that works for you. Even if you cannot sleep the whole time, stay in bed and try to give your body a rest. It is during sleep and rest that you body best removes waste and truly resets itself. This is why many people go to the restroom in the morning, either prior to or after breakfast. This eliminates waste that collected overnight while you were asleep.

Finally, go for a walk each day, preferably in nature and when the sun is shining. A one-to-two mile walk (or jog) and not necessarily more is recommended. Certainly, if you want to walk 4 or 5 miles that is fine. Do not engage in any rigorous or strenuous exercise for the three days. Yoga stretches, Tai Chi and walking are permitted. However, give your body a rest from any intensive workout routine and let it reset.

The three day starting point is required to cleanse and hydrate the body and to begin the healing process.

4 A HEALTHY LIFESTYLE

The main goal of adopting a healthy lifestyle is to eat and live more naturally and in harmony with nature. Therefore, it is important to get rid of all foods in your kitchen (and home) that are processed and full of preservatives, artificial sweeteners, salts, etc. Replace these items with fruits, vegetables, whole grains, legumes, and nuts and seeds. In re-stocking your kitchen exclude any items that may cause an allergic reaction.

The best foods to eat are made by nature, i.e., whole foods. These food, which include fruits, vegetables, whole grains, legumes, and nuts and seeds, should be eaten every day. Raw as well as cooked foods should be consumed in order to obtain the maximum nutrients for the brain and body. Raw foods are fresh and hydrating so you can consume as much food in raw form as possible. This does not mean that you have to adopt a "fully raw food" diet. If you choose to go "raw only" for a day or for a period of time that is fine. But, for the longer term, cooked foods should also be consumed, especially in the winter months. One of the easiest ways to add raw foods to supplement your daily diet is to start each day with fruit as part of breakfast and a starter salad for lunch and dinner. Raw food snacks such as apples, oranges, tomatoes, cucumbers, celery, carrots, lettuce, etc. are also excellent.

The majority of your meals from this point onward should comprise vegetables, legumes, and nuts and seeds. Some fruits and whole grains should also be consumed regularly. Foods such as meat, fish milk, eggs and cheese are generally not recommended. However, if you do eat these foods, please keep it to a minimum, e.g., eat egg whites occasionally and eat fish once a month or only on special holidays. If milk is desired, select skim milk and consume it only if needed. It is okay to have these things once in awhile, but they should not be consumed regularly. With the availability and ease of making vegan milk, e.g., soy milk, rice milk, almond milk, the use of animal sourced milk can easily be kept to a minimum or eliminated altogether.

To ensure that you are eating a healthy and well-balanced diet, periodically track your food and nutrition intake and confirm that you are meeting all the daily nutritional requirements. Applications that provide such information include, e.g., cronometer, fitday, myfitnesspal, LoseIt, Sparkpeople, and FatSecret. Many of these applications have free web-based tools. Fitness applications can also have wearable devices that interconnect with their application software e.g., a watch, a blood pressure monitor, a digital scale, and can be used to help you in your health journey. There are a plethora of apps and tools that provide this type of information. Maintaining a food journal for a period of time may also help to maintain a steady diet. One way to "journalize" daily food intake is to take a picture of everything you eat so that it can be logged into a system at the end of the day. Your diet should be well-balanced and provide sufficient calories and nutrition to fuel your body. Drink caffeinated coffee and tea sparingly. Most people who drink too much coffee/tea are dehydrated and don't even know it. A good rule of thumb when drinking tea or coffee is to consume an extra glass of water for each such beverage. It is important to hydrate the body. Listen to your body and it will tell you how much food and water it needs.

Based on your food intake, you may need to take supplements daily e.g., Vitamin B12 and Vitamin D. If not eating sufficient calcium rich foods, a calcium supplement (which requires the presence of Vitamin D for optimal absorption) may also be required. In addition, it may be useful to occasionally take a good multivitamin to ensure that your body is not missing any essential nutrients. In particular, if you wish to go on a strict vegan diet, ensure that you are meeting all your nutritional requirements, particularly for Vitamin B12, Vitamin D, Vitamin E, Calcium, Potassium, and the proper ratio of Omega 3 to Omega 6 fatty acids. A DHA supplement (Docosahexaenoic acid) is also recommended as it may also be needed for brain health for the longer term.

The other elements of a healthy lifestyle include clean water, fresh air, sunshine, regular exercise, and sleep. The water should be fresh and clean, preferably from a spring or water that has been filtered. Daily walks to obtain fresh air, sunshine and exercise are recommended. Other forms of exercise are discussed in Chapter 7. It is also crucial to connect with people each day and get sufficient restful sleep each night.

5 THE POWER OF FOOD

Food is an essential building block for health and energy and it deserves priority focus. The food we consume is needed for proper functioning of the body (and brain) and nothing else compares to it—not vitamins, pills or anything that is not real food. Food impacts the human body at the inter and intra-cellular level. It comes into the most intimate contact with the body's internal system and the nutrients it imparts are intended to feed the cells in the body and thereby ensure their proper functioning. This is how important the right food is for health and well being. The wrong food, on the other hand, can wreak havoc in the body. (The same correlation applies to drinks as well.) Consuming the right food is crucial for both physical and mental health.

It is amazing how powerful the right food can be for achieving health. There is no replacement for real food made by nature. The reason is that food in nature is especially made to be eaten my man (and woman) and animals. Exercise is secondary to food in determining health. Over the millions of years of existence, humans and their food have evolved a highly complementary, bio-compatible relationship. It is truly a symbiotic relationship —a marriage made on earth (and possibly in heaven). In reality, what humans eat is what the earth "sows." In the old days, the sowing was done through seed propagation based on what we ate and expelled in our fecal matter. In modern day, for humans, this is accomplished via farming and other food production methods. Humans (like other animals) are designed to propagate plants and seeds based on what we like to eat and what tastes good to us. In this manner we "reap" the food that we love when we "sow" it Sounds like the adage "you reap what you sow" is true, at least at this very basic level of food production.[2]

Our bodies are best fed when we eat food made by nature. Therefore, it is crucial to eat whole fruits, vegetables, whole grains, legumes, and nuts and seeds. The sole purpose of fruits and vegetables is to be eaten. Unlike what one may think, fruits, vegetables are not "killed" in the process of being eaten. On the whole (pun intended), fruits and vegetables benefit from being eaten as this allows their seeds to open up and "spread" to other places where resources may be more abundant. Grains, legumes, and nuts and seeds—which are all seeds—also benefit from being spread across the planet and thus benefit from being eaten. Indeed, some of the seeds that are eaten will not be able to reproduce, but in the process some seeds will make it into the soil and reproduce. This is how nature has designed the system. By eating fruits and vegetables and eating the seeds that we find palatable, we are actually helping the planet to propagate the right fruit and

---

[2] It is also important to note that, prior to human intervention, fruits were not as sweet as they are today. Fruits have been made sweeter as a result of seed selection, hybridization, and other forms of human engineering. Our bodies are designed to eat fruits that were not so sweet. We have made fruits much sweeter. Thus, we have to be careful regarding the quantity and type of fruits we consume on a daily basis.

vegetable bearing plant life throughout the planet. Starting to see similarities between our role and the role of bees that held pollinate flowers? Indeed, we are like the bees. The food that we help propagate is the most suitable food for our bodies and we have a mutually beneficial symbiotic relationship with such foods.

It is important to eat a wide variety of fruits, vegetables, grains and seeds. The reason for consuming a variety of foods is that each fruit, vegetable etc. provides its own set of nutrients and combination of nutrients that benefit the body. Indeed, whole foods, including plants also serve our needs for protein. It may seem surprising, but many natural foods (e. g., greens) contain all the commonly occurring essential amino acids, i.e., the building blocks of proteins needed by the body. Altogether, these nature-made foods provide total nutrition to the body.

The best source of essential nutrients to fuel the body is actual food. Extensive research shows that vitamins and other nutrients in pill form are often insufficient to meet the body's needs. The reason is that real food, offers a host of the micronutrients that interplay (just like an orchestra) to help the body obtain the needed vitamins and minerals. Thus, the pills are insufficient on their own.

The above notwithstanding, over the millennia, the nutritional value of the earth's food supply has been declining. Thus, sometimes supplements may be needed to help meet the body's total nutritional requirements. It is therefore advised that a high quality vitamin and mineral supplement be taken periodically (rather than daily) along with consuming high quality food. It is important to emphasize that multivitamins and supplements consumed should be high quality and should only be taken periodically rather than daily.

Having established the importance of whole food, the question of how of each macronutrient to eat comes up. An individual can actually eat as many fruits and vegetables as they wish. However, based on age, gender, and energy utilization and body requirements, it is essential to eat all food, including fruits and vegetables, in proper proportions. What does this mean? There are estimates of essential macronutrients, i.e., carbohydrates, fats and protein that should be taken by an individual. These estimates can be calculated for a person based on their age, gender and activity level. One excellent source for calculating this information is the United States Institute of Medicine's recommendations outlined on their website (www.nationalacademies.org.). An online calculator such as calculator.net derives information about the suggested daily intake of macronutrients from this Institute of Medicine on the following basis:

Carbohydrates

Based on the effects on risk of heart disease and obesity, the Institute of Medicine recommends that American and Canadian adults get 40% to 65% of their dietary energy from carbohydrates. The Food and Agriculture Organization and the World Health Organization jointly recommend that national dietary guidelines set a goal of 55% to 75% of total energy from carbohydrates, but only 10% directly from sugars (their term for simple carbohydrates).

By definition, carbohydrates are organic compounds that consist only of hydrogen, oxygen, and carbon, with hydrogen and oxygen in the 2:1 ratio. Carbohydrates, protein, and fats are the most important elements for a human being's good nutrition. One gram of carbohydrate contains around 3.75 calories of energy (or 106 calories per ounce). Carbohydrates are broken down and classified into "simple" and "complex" carbohydrates. Foods high in simple carbohydrates include fruits, sugars, sweets, and soft drinks. Foods made mainly from rice, wheat, corn, potatoes, and beans, such as breads, pastas, noodles, etc., are high in complex carbohydrates. Nutritionists generally recommend complex carbohydrates, and nutrient-rich simple carbohydrate food, such as fruit (glucose or fructose) and dairy products (lactose) for the bulk of carbohydrate consumption. Simple sugars, such as candy and sugary drinks, are generally not recommended.

Fats

Controlled intake of some fat is good for health. Normally, saturated fats and trans fats are harmful. Monounsaturated fats, Polyunsaturated fats, and Omega-3 fatty acids are considered to be healthier. The recommended fat intake are listed below.

- Take less than 10% of calories from saturated fats. Less than 7% to further reduce the risk to heart disease.
- Replace solid fats with unsaturated fat if possible.
- Take as little trans fat as possible.
- Take less than 300 mg of dietary cholesterol per day.

Protein

The amount of protein needed daily by human body relies on many conditions. Normally it is estimated based on the body weight (0.8-1.8 gram/kg of body weight), or as a percentage of Total Calories intake (10%-35%), or simply based on age.

Another question that often comes up is whether food should be eaten raw or cooked? Indeed, many foods should be eaten both raw and cooked. For example, cooked carrots and tomatoes offer very high nutrition and perhaps more nutrition when cooked rather than raw. Cooking can also affect the "sugar load" of particular foods. For example, cooked carrots have a higher sugar load as compared with raw carrots. This is fine as long as the nutritional value of the food is not compromised and the cooking is factored in the the calculation of total daily intake of nutrients. Cooking food in a particular manner can impact its nutritional value. For example, boiled regular and sweet potatoes have a higher nutritional value than if they were baked or fried. Keep these aspects of cooking in mind when deciding what to eat cooked and how to cook it.

Another factor to consider is the safety of the food, which is particularly important for individuals with compromised immune systems and the elderly. Ensure that all raw food is carefully washed. The food safety issue applies to all food—cooked and raw. But, when eating raw, it is important to ensure careful washing as heat will not be applied to help fight off the bacteria and other food borne disease causing organisms. One way of increasing the safety of raw food is to wash it using hot water or subjecting raw food to heat for a short period of time.

It is also important to manage food intake throughout the day, i.e., after eating foods/meals that are high carbohydrate, give your body a rest for 2 to 3 hours before consuming additional carbs. Instead, eat something with fat and protein (e.g., some nuts and seeds or celery with a nut butter). An excellent way to give your body a fresh start in the morning is to drink some water or go outside for 10 minutes and let the sun help you wake up. For late night snacking, a protein rich snack (e.g., a few nuts or a nut butter with celery sticks) may help ward off hunger and keep the body satiated while sleeping. Keep these factors in mind and your body will respond with kindness in return. It may seem that there is a lot of work to do to eat in this manner, but once you learn and apply the basic principles, eating like this will become second nature.

For most people, as they age, better regulation of the sugar load placed on the body and the brain becomes crucial. Also, if one is faced with serious illness, managing sugar (and thus carbohydrates) in the body is very important. Current research shows that cancer cells grow faster in the presence of excess sugar. Thus, it is important to control sugar intake. This does not mean that one should not eat sugar/carbohydrates. Carbohydrates (which are the main source of sugar) are actually critical for the human body. All cells, including brain cells, use glucose as the immediate source of energy. However, bombarding the body with sugar is not the answer. Just like too much of anything is not good, at high doses, excess sugar can become "poisonous" and thus detrimental to good health. However, at the proper dosage, it is the perfect means for achieving vigor and energy. Often this means, eating more complex carbohydrates and limiting consumption of simple carbohydrates. If you are insulin resistant or likely to become insulin resistant in the near future, it is best to get into the habit of eating foods that are relatively low (or medium) in glycemic load. This is not as hard as it may seem.[3]

A note regarding fruits. Some people believe that one can consume endless quantities of fruit, e.g., fruitarians. This however does not always apply. Our bodies cannot process endless amounts of carbohydrates, fats or protein.

It is important to not over eat (or under eat) in any one category on a regular basis. In the case of sugar, which is a carbohydrate, unless one is young and very physically active—and thus able to "burn off" the excess sugar—intake of sugar, including from fruit, juices and other source should be carefully managed. Fruit is essentially nature's dessert and should be consumed in this manner—on average 2 or 3 times per day—at a certain point in life. Fruit is a very important aspect of healthy eating and most

---

[3] The glycemic load (GL) of food is a number that estimates how much the food will raise a person's blood glucose level after eating it. One unit of glycemic load approximates the effect of consuming one gram of glucose.[1] Glycemic load accounts for how much carbohydrate is in the food and how much each gram of carbohydrate in the food raises blood glucose levels. Glycemic load is based. Source: Wikipedia.

fruits are loaded with nutrients. However, once an individual becomes insulin resistant, they need to watch how much fruit, and, more generally, total daily intake of carbohydrates and fats. Having said this, fruit is very good for human health so don't shy away from fruit; instead, just manage its intake and select more low sugar and high fiber fruits such as raspberries, blackberries, pears, and green apples, etc. Fat intake is also critical for health, but the total daily fat intake needs to be carefully managed. In particular, saturated fats and trans fats consumption should be limited. Protein is a very important macronutrient as well. However, regular overconsumption of protein carries serious consequences. The proper balance of macronutrients in whole food form is essential for health.

It is also essential manage salt intake (i.e., sodium chloride). Sodium chloride impacts the osmotic pressure of cells. The body gets rid of excess salt by flushing it out with water. There is a maximum concentration of salt to water that the kidneys are able to manage. The kidneys cannot concentrate pure salt to remove it from the body; instead, they require excess water to get rid of it. This is yet another reason to cut out preserved foods as most preserved foods have a relatively high salt content thus one needs to drink sufficient water to maintain kidney health. Certainly, salt is important, and in low quantities it is good for you. It should be noted that salt is found naturally occurring, in low concentration, in some vegetables, e.g., swiss chard, celery, bell peppers, carrots, artichoke, broccoli, sweet potatoes, and radishes Thus, the need for added salt is much lower than what most people consume.

It is important to eat foods that are palatable and offer satiety. Thus, if desired, salt cooked vegetables a little so that they taste good rather than not eating them. An alternative to using excess salt is to use lemon juice to enhance the flavor of food. Lemon is an excellent salt substitute. In addition, use a host of spices and herbs to enhance the flavor of food and make it much more palatable. Eat whole foods that you like. It may take a while for your taste buds to adjust, but eventually they will tell you which whole foods are appealing.

Daily intake of fiber and starch, particularly resistant starch, is recommended. According to the United States Institute of Medicine, the recommended intake for total fiber for adults 50 years and younger is set at 38 grams for men and 25 grams for women, while for men and women over 50 it is 30 and 21 grams per day, respectively, due to decreased food consumption. Research shows that societies that eat a high fiber diet and one that is rich in resistant starch are healthier.

How often should you eat and which meals are more important? This is a very important question. The bottom line is one should have a regular meal schedule. All three meals are important. On the other hand, it is also important to give your stomach and digestive system time to process the food and extract nutrients. Thus, give your system a rest for 2 to 3 hours after a full meal. This does not mean that snacks are out of the question. To the contrary having a small snack such as fresh fruit, cucumber, carrot or celery slices, or a handful of nuts, in between meals is an excellent practice. It is important to balance blood sugar and snacks are helpful in achieving this balance. The point is not to eat all day long and instead give the digestive system time to digest the food. Also, do not skip meals on a regular basis. Its best to nourish the body and brain on a regular basis.

Another approach for maintaining a healthy body and losing fat is to intermittently fast. It is not recommended that anyone engage in a long term fast without medical supervision. There is however a logical basis for fasting as humans like other animals have evolved to benefit from intermittent fasting. Many times our ancestors did not find food for a day, or for a few weeks. They also did to have access to the full complement of vitamins and minerals each and every day. Thus, we like other creatures have evolved to sustain ourselves in times of food shortages.

Some research even suggests that intermittent fasting can extend a individual's life. More recently, the findings indicate that, in particular, restricting protein is the reason that fasting is beneficial for the body. Thus, one alternative to fasting is to restrict protein intake periodically.

In modern times, humans have much more access to food. Nevertheless, fasting is a means to give the body a break and allow it to reset. The best way to benefit from fasting is to occasionally skip a meal or two, e.g., if there is no healthy food nearby or you are at a party and there is nothing truly healthy to eat then fasting is recommended. This does not mean that after skipping a meal one should overeat. Instead, the fast should be used to lower the overall food and calorie intake for that day.

Alternatively, one can achieve increased fat loss by increasing and decreasing consumption of calories from day to day while ensuring that daily nutrient need are met. Maintaining a constant, relatively low calorie consumption level each day may not be the best idea as the body adapts and adjusts. Fluctuate the amount of food consumed from one day to the other to keep your body and digestive system active. If you end up eating a lot one day, then scale back the next day or vice versa. The end goal is to maximize nutrient quality while reducing inflammation in the body and ensuring that the hormones and organ systems are active, balanced and functioning properly. The secrets presented in this book are aimed at helping you meet this important goal.

Some of the best food advice that will trigger your journey into health is presented below:

1. Use unsaturated fats to increase good cholesterol (HDL) and reduce inflammation. This requires eliminating processed foods as such foods contain saturated fats as they resist rancidity and are more solid at room temperature. Unsaturated fats include:
    * Extra virgin olive oil
    * Hemp oil
    * Flax oil (high in ligans)

- Canola oil
- Pumpkin seed oil
- Avocados
- Nuts

2. Food to emphasize
   - Fruits -berries and pineapple
   - Dark leafy green vegetables
   - Walnuts
   - Maitake mushrooms
   - Onions and garlic
   - Legumes
   - Spices, including ginger and turmeric

3. Consume high ORAC (Oxygen Radical Absorbance Capacity, which is a measure of food's antioxidant capacity) foods daily, such as berries, kiwi, grapefruit, pomegranates.

4. Protein
   - Plants contain all the essential amino acids that the body need.
   - Plant protein is better than animal protein for the human body.

5. Avoid / Restrict
   - Meat, eggs and dairy
   - Caffeine
   - Alcohol (if drinking alcohol occasionally) red wine is recommended as it contains Resveratrol.

6 THE ELIXIR OF LIFE

Water is the elixir of life. It comprises a significant portion of our bodies, i.e., from 55 to 60 percent for adults on average. Although, the actual percentage varies by individual. Indeed, our cells and organs need adequate water to function properly.[4] Hydrating your body will not only make you feel better, it may alleviate a host of medical issues and allow for healthy weight reduction. Having said this, it is not advisable to drink too much water. We are like other things in nature, if we are not sufficiently hydrated, our skin looses suppleness and if over hydrated we can "drown" in too much water.

How much water is needed each day? According to the US Geological Survey (USGS), the recommended daily intake varies by age and gender. Generally, an adult male needs about 3 liters per day while an adult female needs

---

[4] According to H.H. Mitchell, Journal of Biological Chemistry 158, the brain and heart are composed of 73% water, and the lungs are about 83% water. The skin contains 64% water, muscles and kidneys are 79%, and even the bones are watery: 31%.

about 2.2 liters per day. Some of the daily requirement for water is met by consuming water-rich food, e.g, lettuce watermelon, grapes and apples contain some water. The USGS states that water serves a number of essential functions to keep us all going:

- It is a vital nutrient to the life of every cell, acts first as a building material.
- It regulates our internal body temperature by sweating and respiration.
- It metabolizes and transports, in the blood stream, the carbohydrates and proteins that our bodies use as food.
- It assists in flushing waste mainly through urination.
- It acts as a shock absorber for brain, spinal cord, and fetus; forms saliva ad lubricates the joints.

Proper hydration is crucial for health and to keep the organs running efficiently and effectively. For example, adequate hydration may reduce the incidence of kidney stones. The American College of Physicians has established new guidelines to help patients who are prone to kidney stones to reduce their risk for developing them again in the future. A key piece of advice is to drink at least two liters of water or other fluids a day. Research has found that drinking more fluids could cut the chances of recurrent kidney stones by at least half. "The reason that water is supposedly helpful is that it is a mechanical flushing process so that stone fragments can pass but also so the urine doesn't sediment in the kidney and collect."[5]

Hydration can be in the form of water, fruits, vegetables, smoothies, soups etc. Start each day with a glass or two of water to jumpstart your system. The key point is to ensure that your body has enough fluids. As mentioned earlier, this does not mean that more is better. Over-

---

[5] Dr. Elizabeth Kavaler, "New guidelines could cut risk of kidney stones," CBS News.

hydration is not the goal and can be very harmful. The best approach is to drink water daily, eat whole foods, and take in liquids. Listen to your body and you will become attuned to knowing when you need to hydrate. Some early signs of dehydration include dryness at the edges of the lips or the lip line, dry skin, and dry hair.

In terms of foods containing water, smoothies can indeed be added to the diet. Juices and other sweet drinks on the other hand should be consumed sparingly. If possible, eliminate juices altogether. If taking juice as a regular part of your diet, please make sure the juice is low in sugar and salt. Consumption of caffeinated tea and coffee should also be limited. Herbal teas are fine. For example, a cup of green tea daily is actually good for health. This does not mean that one can never have juice, or coffee or tea. To the contrary, perhaps a cup or two of coffee or tea is part of a regimen. That is fine just as long as one does not overdo it and drinks sufficient water to counteract the dehydration effect. The goals here is to get as clean a diet as possible while allowing for situations were these types of drinks (and foods) are okay to consume. It is recommended that after drinking caffeinated drinks, drink an extra a glass of water as these drinks are dehydrating.

7 EXERCISE REGIMEN

It is important to stay physically active throughout life. The importance of staying active needs to be underscored. All creatures that are meant to move (motile) benefit from movement. Unlike trees, plants, grasses etc., which are not designed to move, motile organisms are meant to move. Thus, motile organisms benefit from movement. It does not have to be constant movement, but rather periodic movement. As you may be aware, people who are on the go all the time are slimmer, and they have fewer problems such as constipation, etc. Bottom line, humans benefit from regular movement.

Movement is not needed simply to burn off calories. Its role is much broader. In addition to burning calories, movement helps to: maintain skeletal muscle activity (which improves skeletal muscle insulin sensitivity); strengthen bones, improve oxygenation of the body; promote bodily flow (inflow of nutrients and oxygen and outflow of waste/toxins and carbon dioxide); promote the energy production cycle at the cellular level; and, release cortisol to reduce stress Unquestionably, it is important to remain physically active throughout life. Movement is as important as food and water for survival. One of the reasons that the health of older individuals declines precipitously is that they stop moving as much, which compromises their health and accelerates aging.

Staying active is the key to survival in the modern day. If we don't move we encounter a host of issues, including the possibility of blood clots and death. As humans, we have to remain both mentally and physically active. Our brains and bodies need exercise. This does not mean that being active all the time is the best for health. To the contrary, the goal is to achieve a healthy and active lifestyle coupled with adequate rest and relaxation. Similarly, our brains need to remain active and alert but the brain also benefits from rest and relaxation. Our bodies and brain also require adequate sleep to function properly.

An exercise regimen of 4 to 5 times a week is recommended. The regimen can include walking, gardening, tai chi, bicycling, hiking, tennis, group sports, playing with children, dancing, yoga, etc. One can also choose to run, jog, lift weights, or engage in any other form of exercise. In the end, exercise benefits the body and the mind. As we age, it is even more important to stay active in order to promote blood flow (including to the brain) and maintain muscle strength. Leading a sedentary lifestyle only leads to problems. So, find things you like to do and make it a habit to stay active. To offer an example, one person who lived a very long life revealed that he walked and did light exercises every day and when he got over 100 years old and was unable to walk, he would do about 100 bicycle exercises with his legs while laying in bed. He knew the importance of movement and found a way to move even as he got very old. As noted by this example, what is needed is periodic movement (and not necessarily high impact exercise) to maintain health.

It is important to exercise regularly but not to overdo it. As mentioned, the exercise does not have to rigorous. It can be as simple as gardening or walking. It is best when the activity involves multiple muscle groups and is pleasurable and tension releasing. Sweating while exercising is also beneficial as it allows an individual to cool down and it releases toxins. Too much exercise is not recommended as it adds undue stress to the body and lead to oxidative stress. Excessive exercise can weaken the immune system, it can lead to breakdown of muscles and organ systems and throw the body's hormones off kilter— e.g., it can lead to abnormal rhythm of the heart, artery wall stiffing, patchy scarring of the heart and it can even cause kidney failure The goal is to strike the right balance in order to reaps the benefits of movement.

There are a range of physical activities and exercises in which one can engage. According to the National Institute on Aging at the National Institute of Heath, exercise and physical activity fall into four main categories—endurance, strength, balance, and flexibility. Most people tend to focus on one activity or one type of activity and think they're doing enough. However, each type of activity is different and doing them all offers the most benefits.

The four main categories of physical activity are:

1. **Endurance** activities focus on increasing heart rate and breathing and include fast walking, dancing, tennis, soccer, basketball, yard work etc.

2. **Strength** exercises focus on maintaining (or increasing) muscle strength. These include resistances and weight bearing exercises.

3. **Balance** exercises help prevent falls. These exercises are particularly important as people age. Many lower-body strength exercises also will improve balance. They include standing on one foot, heel-to-toe movement and walking, and Tai Chi.

4. **Flexibility** exercises stretch your muscles and can help your body stay limber. Flexibility is important as exercise can make muscles tight and aging makes an individual staff. Flexibility gives

you more freedom of movement for other exercises as well as for your everyday activities. Exercises that increase flexibility include shoulder and upper arm stretches, calf stretches, and yoga.

Exercises is not just for the physically fit; it is important for everyone to move, to flex and strengthen their muscles, and maintain balance. Exercises are best done outdoors, in fresh air and sunshine. However, going to a gym is better than not exercising at all. If exercising in a gym, take time out for walks or sit outdoors.

If you are unable to go to a gym or exercise elsewhere, whether it is because of weight, health, disability or other reasons, there are some "home-based" alternatives to consider:

1. **Endurance** activities could include walking around the house certain number of times per day or walking up and down the stairs, or doing jump rope and jumping jacks. If one is physically disabled, e.g., in a wheelchair and using a walker or a cane, focus on slow walking if possible. Else, engage in simple exercises such as toe touches, shifting your body from side to side, marching in place while sitting or standing, and standing up and sitting down multiple times while using a support such as a walker or a cane.

2. **Strength** exercises include using small weights such as bags of dry beans/legumes or bottles filled with water as weights. One can also use heavier weights and also add ankle weights. If necessary, strength exercises can be done while sitting.

3. **Balance** exercises can be done anywhere. One can sit in a chair and do heel-toe movements repetitiously. Yoga also offers many balancing postures which can be done anywhere, including while brushing teeth, cooking meals or flying in a

airplane (yes the small open hallway area can be used on a long distance to do exercises).

4. **Flexibility** exercises include arm and shoulder stretches, toe touches etc. One can even try to move individual muscles while sitting and making small muscle movements all over their body. Massaging arms and legs is also a form of movement. Doors, walls, hand towels can be used for resistance to stretch arms, shoulders, legs, chest, and back. Sitting on the floor (or a carpet or pillow) while watching a movie can also increase flexibility.

The body is like a giant, flowing river—if the blood flow is maintained then the body is able to move nutrients to the cells and organ systems and remove toxins out of the body. Else, the body becomes still and unable to operate effectively. Staying active is the key to keep the river in the body flowing. This does not mean extensive exercise. Too much exercise can lead to oxidative stress just as the river can overflow due to floods. The key is to move with conviction, flex the muscles to keep them strong and flexible, and relieve stress in the process.

8 CARBOHYDRATES, FATS AND PROTEIN

Imagine proteins as the frame of a vehicle, fats as the upholstery and features that make it durable, and carbohydrates as the fuel to power and drive the machine.

When considering dieting, bodybuilding or reviewing a health regimen, often the topic of carbohydrates, fats and proteins comes up. Indeed these three macronutrients are important for sustenance. The question is what to consume, what macronutrients are important and how much of each of these macronutrients is needed for proper functioning of the body. The good news is that the human body is very adept at utilizing all of these macronutrients. So, how does the human body work?

The basics of how the body uses these macronutrients is that if all three macronutrients are abundant in one's diet, carbohydrates and fats will be used to generate energy while proteins will be used to build muscles and serve other purposes such as forming the basis for hormone production etc. If there is a shortage of carbohydrates and fats, proteins will be used to generate energy. If all three are in short supply, protein from muscles will be extracted and used for energy generation. Thus, on a long term basis, all these macronutrients are required for proper functioning of the human body.

Carbohydrates are the easiest source of energy for the body to utilize and the human body can only store excess carbohydrates for a day or two. Excess carbohydrates are stored in the form of glucose in the liver and if there is leftover glucose, it is stored as glycogen or fat in the liver. Thus, when carbohydrates are scarce, the stored glucose and glycogen can be used to provide energy to the body.

Fats are broken down into fatty acids which then serve as an energy source for the body. Excess fatty acids are stored as triglycerides in fat cells, which have unlimited storage capacity. There is, however, one part of the human body, the brain, that cannot generate energy from fatty acids. The brain runs on glucose and if there is insufficient glucose, the body generates ketones for the brain's energy requirements.

Protein from food is broken down in the human body into amino acids, which are then used to build new protein and to perform various other functions. As mentioned earlier, in the absence of carbohydrates and fat, protein can be used to generate energy. At some point, if needed, protein from muscle can be extracted and used to generate energy. If this happens, it is knows as "muscle wastage" which is not good in the long run.

What is the ideal ratio of carbohydrates, fats and protein for the human body? There is no ideal diet with the perfect ratio of carbohydrates, fats and proteins that fits everyone at every age. However, there are some basic requirements that must be met by the body and moderation is recommended. For example, the moderate carbohydrate approach to dieting calls for eating whole fruits, whole vegetables, and whole grains and legumes to the extent possible and limiting refined carbohydrates. This is because whole foods not only contain fiber that slows down the process of breaking down the food for energy generation, they also contain the complement of micronutrients needed by the body to meet its nutritional needs. The benefits of this diet is that the body gets the good carbohydrates and limits the bad carbohydrates.

The main message is that unless medically necessary do not restrict carbohydrates, especially whole food sourced carbohydrates, severely as they are the primary energy source for the body. Similarly, fats are crucial for the body for performing certain functions and some micronutrients are "fat soluble" meaning that they require the presence of fat to be utilized. Thus, fats should also be consumed daily. The best form of fat is unsaturated and whole sourced, e.g., from nuts and seeds, avocados, etc. Protein is also essential for the body and should ideally be plant sourced as plant protein is better for the human body than animal sourced protein.[6] Meat and animal-based products are common sources of protein in today's world, but an individual can get the full complement of amino acids that comprise proteins from plant sources. It may seem surprising but many whole plant foods contain protein. Though it takes some planning, protein can be found in certain fruits, vegetables, grains, legumes, and nuts and seeds. Protein from these sources comes without the highly saturated fats and other issues (e.g., pus found in milk and viruses found in meat) that accompany meat and other animal products. For example, proteins are found in most leafy green vegetables and a host of other vegetables. Seeds and nuts are excellent source of plant protein as well.

What is important is to ensure proper intake of foods that provide the necessary nutrients while limiting overconsumption. The best way to accomplish this is to determine the proper ratio of carbohydrates, fats and protein for your age, gender and size and logging in your

---

[6] Gregor, Michael, M.D.., and Stone, Gene, *How Not to Die*, MacMillan Children's Publishing, 2015.

food intake periodically to ensure that the full set of nutrients in the proper ratios are being consumed on a regular basis.

Regarding the question of proper ratio of carbohydrates, fats, and protein, there is some variation between individuals, by age, by gender and other factors. As discussed in Chapter 5, one can estimate the carbohydrate, fat, and protein they should consumed based on their age, gender and activity level using an online calculator such as calculator.net. In the end, it is not just about getting the right quantity of carbohydrates, fats, and proteins, the kinds of foods consumed to obtain these macronutrients matters a lot.

9 COMPARATIVE REVIEW OF DIETS

A brief comparative review of the various diets and their pros and cons are presented in this chapter. The diet for a svelte and healthy body is also presented along with the supporting rationale.

Atkins Diet

The Atkins Diet, put forward by Dr. Atkins, who was a cardiologist, is a low carbohydrate, high fat diet. This diet focuses on limiting consumption of carbohydrates so the body can burn fat, including body fat, for fuel. This diet works, at least initially, as it reduces the high sugar load on the body and replaces it with protein. The diet focuses on consuming high levels of meat, butter, cheese, eggs etc., which provide protein and fat, in place of carbohydrates. In the absence of carbohydrates, the body burns fat and yields weight loss for a period of time.

Initially, weight loss results as protein and fat replace carbohydrates. However, over time, the body gets burdened with high levels of saturated fat and protein. This leads to a number of diseases such as gout, high cholesterol, diabetes, heart disease, hypertension, stroke, etc. If the carbohydrate intake is measurably reduced, the diet also results in a loss of energy over time. Low carbohydrate diets also reduce blood flow to the heart.[7] According to research in recent years, eating a low carbohydrate is similar to fasting and starvation of the body. The body can operate in starvation mode for a short period of time, but not for the long run. This diet leads to a number of health issues as listed above. Thus, this diet is not recommended as a long term solution.

Ketogenic Diet

The ketogenic diet was originally developed to deal with difficult to control epileptic seizure in children. As mentioned in Chapter 8, ketone bodies generated by the body in the absence of carbohydrates serve as an alternative fuel, in place of glucose, for the brain and thus help mitigate seizures. This diet is similar to the Atkins Diet or the Low Carbohydrate, High Fat (LCHF) diet. The main difference between strict LCHF and the ketogenic diet is that protein is restricted a bit more in this latter diet.

Despite the clear benefits afforded by the ketogenic

---

[7] Dr. Richard Fleming, "an accomplished nuclear cardiologist, enrolled 26 people into a comprehensive study of the effects of diet on cardiac function using the latest in nuclear imaging technology--so-called SPECT scans, enabling him to actually directly measure the blood flow within the coronary arteries." Those patients which followed the healthy vegetarian diet "showed a reversal of their heart disease as expected. Their partially clogged arteries literally got cleaned out. They had 20% less atherosclerotic plaque in their arteries at the end of the year than at the beginning." The health of those patients that followed a low-carb, high-animal protein diet "significantly worsened." Scans showed they had "40 to 50% more artery clogging at the end of the year."

diet, particularly for children who experience seizures, there are clear and dire consequences as result of the high fat intake for all individuals.. Our experience with this diet is limited in that it could not be pursued for an extended period of time due the negative side effects caused by the very high fat content of the diet. The issues that arise on this diet include lack of energy, gastrointestinal stress, hormonal imbalance and a host of other maladies. This diet is thus not recommended as a long term solution.

Paleo Diet

The Paleo Diet is based on eating foods that comprised the human diet during the Paleolithic Era, which was prior to the development of food agriculture.[8] It mimics the diet of hunter gathers and thus limits the use of processed foods, sugar and salt. The diet shuns grains, legumes and dairy products and focuses instead on nuts, meat, etc. The diet is based on high protein, high fiber, moderate to high fat (particularly mono saturated fat) and low carbohydrate foods.

There are some merits associated with this diet given that processed foods, sugar and salt—which are all culprits —are restricted, high fiber is added to the diet, and saturated fat is restricted. This diet also gets people interested in cooking their own food as processed foods are not part of the diet. However, over time, the low carbohydrate levels can reduce energy levels. The high protein intake can lead to issues such as gout and increased likelihood of other diseases. As mentioned earlier, low carb diets also reduce blood flow in the body and eating a low carbohydrate is similar to fasting and starvation of the body. Thus, this diet is not recommended as long term

---

[8] According to Wikipedia, The Paleolithic Era, "...extends from the earliest known use of stone tools, probably by Homo habilis initially, 2.6 million years ago, to the end of the Pleistocene around 10,000 BP."

solution for health and wellness.

Moderate Carbohydrate Diet

The Moderate Carbohydrate diet, as noted in its name, calls for moderation of carbohydrates, i.e., not low carbohydrates and not high carbohydrates. This is a step in the right direction for consumption of carbohydrates, which provide energy to the body and enhance blood flow. The moderation of carbohydrates also limits excess storage of carbohydrates in muscle tissue in the form of glycogen.

However, the diet offers limited information and instead focuses on consuming moderate amounts of carbohydrates to sustain the energy level in the body. This goal is excellent. However, it is important that a healthy diet cover all major macronutrients (and micronutrients) and provide more substantial information to form a healthy daily regimen. This diet appears to focus on the importance of carbohydrates, which is beneficial, but it is unclear if moderating carbohydrates alone is the pathway to health and fitness.

Vegetarian Diet

The vegetarian diet encompasses two variants: (a) the lacto-vegetarian diet, which, in addition to fruits, vegetables, grains, legumes, and nuts and seeds, supports the consumption of cheese and dairy products; and (b) the ovo-lacto vegetarian diet, which supports the consumption of eggs as well as cheese and dairy products.

The benefits of this diet is that it limits protein intake, particularly the consumption of animal protein, and focus on eating a multitude of healthy foods. The problem, however, is that many vegetarians find it hard to lose weight under this diet and instead gain weight. This is likely due to consumption of too many (and the wrong kind of) carbohydrates and fats; particularly grains in the form of white bread, pasta, rice, etc which are not healthy in large quantities. Some vegetarians also eat too much fat in the form of nuts, seeds, butter and cheese. In addition, some vegetarians eat a lot of processed and fried food and use too much oil and butter. Although some vegetarians get healthier on this diet, particularly if they focus on eating whole foods, many continue to have health issues and have difficulty losing weight. This diet also poses challenges for those fighting cancer due to the high levels of carbohydrates consumed. Cancer feeds on sugar and a high carbohydrate diet generates excess sugar. Therefore, this is not an ideal diet for the long term.

Vegan Diet

The Vegan Diet focuses on eating fruits, vegetables, grains, legumes, and nuts and seeds. All foods of animal origin, e.g., honey, are excluded. Most vegans are very conscious of what they eat and how their food is prepared. Some vegans even chose to follow a raw food diet. Strict vegans, in particular animal rights activists, also do not use products derived from animals such as leather, silk, etc.

The vegan diet is considered to be an extreme diet and many find it hard to maintain it on a long term basis. It is too restrictive and challenging to follow. The diet restrict processed foods and it restricts c foods that are ingredients is many dishes (e.g., eggs found in bread). The MEDs (meat, eggs and dairy) are ingredients in many foods consumed in the home and outside the home. Thus, it can be very hard to find foods that meet the requirements of the diet. In addition, the diet focuses attention on fruits and vegetables (and, according to many dieters, there not enough good tasting recipes for vegetables cooked with vegan ingredients). The diet provides sufficient carbohydrates for the body; however, if the consumption of carbohydrates is too high, weight gain and a host of other maladies can arise (yes, an individual can gain weight on a strict vegan diet quite easily). The diet also raises the question of meeting daily nutrient requirements, particularly for Vitamin B12 and Omega 3. Nevertheless, when followed correctly, the diet increases overall energy levels and health outcomes. Most people following this diet generally lose weight and improve their health status over time.

Fruitarian Diet

This diet, which is a subset of the vegan diet, focuses on primarily eating fruits supplemented with some seeds, nuts and vegetables. This is a high carbohydrate, low fat and low protein diet wherein about 80 percent of the diet consists of carbohydrates while the remaining 20 percent consists of fats and protein. Some fruitarians eat a strictly raw food diet, but most individuals on this diet consume both raw and cooked foods.

On this diet, many individuals initially lose weight, particularly those eating raw. Eventually, however, some of these individuals gain it all back. Our experience with this diet has been not only weight gain, but rather a host of issues such as tooth decay and tooth loss, fatty liver disease, pre-diabetes, etc. Over time, the body is unable to manage the high levels of sugar consumed on a regular basis, i.e., unless the individual is very physically active and is able to burn off the sugar before an excess amount is stored in the body. The raw food fruitarians fare a bit better that those eating cooked food, but many fruitarians eventually experience excessive tooth decay and tooth loss. For these and sundry reasons, the fruitarian is not the ideal diet for health.

Healthy Body Diet

Which diet is the right one? Which diet results in better weight management and health management. The diet consumed is critically important but true health also depends on how the food is prepared. It also matters that the body's nutritional requirements, including requirement for fiber, are met on a regular basis, and that hormones and pesticides in the food supply are kept to a minimum.

Eating a plant and fiber rich diet, which is the "vegevore" diet, is the best way forward. Under this diet, eating vegetables is the main goal. Eat whole plant foods that taste good to you. Your palette may need to be cleansed and the taste buds may need to be retrained. But, eventually, the taste buds will reawaken. Remember that cutting out (or cutting down gradually if its too hard to do so immediately) the MEDs (Meat, Eggs, and Dairy) alone limits the amount of hormones, pesticides, radiation etc. entering your body. Fiber in the diet provides magic by helping to build the gut biome that can feed the body and defend it against toxins.

All the major macronutrients found in whole foods are needed by the body to maintain growth and to repair the body. This is among the reasons that this diet works. When eating carbohydrates, especially, whole food sourced carbohydrates, think of energy. These types of carbohydrates are the "fuel" for running the body and the daily fuel requirement should be met in order for the body to run correctly. But, if consuming too many carbohydrates for the level of activity, then the carbohydrates become a poison to the system over time. Think of sustenance when considering fats. Fats should ideally be whole sourced and primarily unsaturated. Eaten in the right proportion, fats offer satiety and an easy approach to storing energy. However, consuming too much fat, particularly too much saturated fat, can be a very fast way to poison to the system. Protein should also be whole and plant sourced ideally. Though many may not realize it, a number of foods made by nature include protein. Protein forms the foundation of our bodies; it comprises, our bones, muscles, arteries and veins, skin, hair, finger and toe nails, etc. Protein is found abundantly in leafy greens, legumes, and nuts and seeds.

In the end, it is about achieving the right balance for the body, depending on one's age, gender, height, weight, level of activity, etc. The "vegevore" diet, which is a plant and fiber strong diet, is the basis for building a svelte and healthy body. In terms of food preparation, the goals is to reduce advanced glycation end produts (AGEs) in food. This can be best accomplished maintaining a plant strong whole food diet and by cooking plants/vegetables using minimal and slow cooking methods at low temperatures. Cooking with acids such as vinegar and lemon juice is also considered beneficial. Finally, it is important to ensure that your body is obtaining its full complement of macro and micro nutrients. Give this diet a chance; in return, the body will respond in amazing ways.

10 DIGESTION

The health and diet secrets presented in this book lead to excellent health. It is not the diet pills and elixirs, nor the Atkins, the ketogenic, the paleolithic, the vegetarian, the vegan, the fruitarian and host of other diets, that yield health alone. There is not any one strict diet alone that works. Its a way of eating and living that culls the knowledge gleamed from the various diets and lifestyles in the proper way that activates a healthy and beautiful body.

In my case, it was focusing on whole foods, staying away from gluten (due to celiac), keeping the carbohydrate load in check, maintaining plant-based fat and protein sources, treating fruit as nature's dessert, staying hydrated, maintaining an active lifestyle, and maintaining a connection with nature. In the process of cleaning my diet and lifestyle regimen, I learned something that Grandmas around the world have been saying for centuries: "Eat your fiber." Grandma was right after all. Eat high fiber fruits and vegetables. If humans focus on eating whole foods that are high in both nutrition and fiber, this will lead to increased health and energy.

Fiber does much more than add bulk to the diet. It is

important for inhibiting bad bacteria and promoting good bacteria in the digestive system. It acts as a prebiotic to keep the host of gut bacteria in balance. The gut is considered to be the second brain of the body and thus keeping the gut biome healthy is critical. Fiber is also important for nutrient absorption and for stimulating colonic flow. Fiber slows down the release of nutrients and minerals such that the body can manage it best—it is nature's s time-release system (just like a time release capsule) for nourishing the body and the brain on a continuous basis. Always remember to consume a large percentage of high fiber foods each day. It is important to consume natural fiber found in food rather than using extracted fiber such as Metamucil, i.e., if possible. There are a combination of nutrients in whole foods that work with natural fiber that are important for digestion as well as health and energy. Foods high in fiber are naturally low in carbohydrates, which keeps diabetes and other health issues at bay. Fiber also wins as it helps keep an individual feel satiated.

One way to check that your diet is high fiber is to ensure that it results in fast digestion, i.e., the length of time that food stays in your system should be short (but not unusually short as with diarrhea). Stated in another way, fiber enables your body to absorb nutrients from food and expel fecal matter and toxins in a timely manner. If you are eating the right foods this should not be a problem. It may take some time to get there, but this should not be an issue with the right diet. Eating high fiber foods should help increase energy levels as the body is better fed and clean, on a continuous basis. The only issue that may arise is that your digestion becomes so efficient that, when nature calls, you may need to find a bathroom relatively quickly. There is no doubt that a high fiber, nutrient-rich diet will lead to increased energy as well as fast digestion.

According to Anish Sheth, MD, co-author of the books *What's Your Poo Telling You?* and *What's My Pee Telling*

Me?, water comprises about 75 percent of your bowel movements. The rest is an combination of "fiber, dead and live bacteria, other cells, and mucus. Soluble fibers found in foods like beans and nuts are broken down during digestion and form a gel-like substance that becomes part of your poop." Do you hit the bathroom at the same exact time every morning, or can you go days before you need to go No. 2? It's all normal, says Sheth— the important thing is that you're consistent for your own routine. A big decrease in output could be due to a diet change (fiber intake), which is why many people find they're less regular on weekends or vacation—they may be eating less fiber or working out less often, both of which promote healthy digestion. Other factors affecting output —either a decrease or an increase—are gastrointestinal disorders, an overactive thyroid, or colon cancer.

Another advocate of looking before you flush is Mehmet Oz, MD, host of *The Dr. Oz Show*, who explained during a now-famous appearance on The Oprah Winfrey Show that the perfect stool is log-like and S-shaped, not broken up into pieces. Part of getting that log-style shape, compared to poo that comes out more pebbly-looking, comes from eating fiber as it lends bulk to stool and acts as a glue to keep the stool stuck together as it exits your body. Pencil-thin poops, on the other hand, can be a sign of rectal cancer, which narrows the opening through which stool passes, according to Seth.

Cultural differences play a role too. Sheth notes in his book that South Asians unload nearly three times as much stool as British people do, a difference he explains is largely due to the higher fiber content in their diet.

According to Sheth on his website DrStool.com states that the average American man excretes 150 grams (about one-third of a pound) of stool every day, or the equivalent of 5 tons in a lifetime. Most of the time, a diet devoid of fiber, which keeps your bowels regular and prevents constipation and hard stools, is to blame. Most Americans eat 10 to 15 grams of fiber a day; doctors recommend 30 to 35 grams to prevent hemorrhoids, according to researchers from Los Angeles Medical Center.

11 MAKING DIETARY CHANGES: ADDRESSING CONCERNS

$\mathbf{F}$ood and health are intimately linked. Food provides the body with the necessary nutrients to provide energy to the body, to maintain it, and to defend the body from toxins and foreign agents. In this sense, food serves as a vital life force for the body.

Individuals who go on various diets are well intended, but they do not always understand the intimate relationship that exists between food and health. Their goal is often to lose weight, but without focusing on health they cannot be successful. Follower of all diets can place their health at risk if they do not understand this relationship. Those who consume too much and overeat experience health risks as well. To be specific, even individuals who are vegetarians, vegans and fruitarians can be at risk of not consuming a balanced and nutritious diet. For example, consuming too many carbohydrates and fats, teenaged and children can display symptoms of early onset diabetes and possibly asthma. Consuming too few carbohydrates and instead consuming high levels of protein and fat, particularly animal-based protein, can lead to early onset of heart disease, reduce blood flow and energy in the body. The absence of Vitamin D, which can be absorbed through proper sun exposure or through supplements, can lead to dental and skeletal fragility. So, what is the path to health? It is to understand the relationship between food and the body and the relationship between food and the gut biome and eat accordingly. Based on this understanding, one of the best ways to achieve health is to eat a whole food, plant and fiber rich diet and periodically track food intake to ensure a proper nutritional profile.

Children and teenagers who go on such diets without sufficient knowledge about food and nutrition are particularly at risk. Their bodies are growing and transforming and their require proper nutrition else they face negative health consequences. They need to ensure that they are taking all the essential macronutrients and micronutrients in the proper proportions from food and lifestyle choices, and if not through vitamin supplements. Being a teenager can be stressful and the desire for a good body image can override heath interests.

Teenagers in particular lead busy lives and can easily forget to eat properly. They are also undergoing body transformations and dealing with hormonal changes and without a proper diet, they can compromise their health relatively quickly. This is the reason many parents are reluctant to allow their children and teenagers to follow various diets. The best way a young individual interested in following a particular diet can achieve success (and allay parental concerns) is to log their food intake daily and show their parents that they are following a healthy diet.

Adults following various diets can experience issues as well. For example, a very high carbohydrate diet can lead to diabetes and fatty liver disease. It can also exacerbate asthma and feed cancer. This is quite true. So, maintaining a log to ensure proper nutrition is essential for anyone interested in a svelte and healthy body.

12 REST AND RELAXATION

During rest and relaxation, and particularly during sleep, the body rejuvenates and resets itself. During sleep, the also body gets rid of toxins most efficiently. It is also during sleep that dieters shed excess body weight. Sufficient sleep on a regular basis is required for healthy weight loss. The importance of sleep cannot be sufficiently underscored. A good sleep is "free" so take advantage of it. It is a very precious gift that we should not take lightly. Too much sleep is also not good. Its a matter of getting the right amount of sleep consistently. In addition to night time sleep, it is important to relax and engage in deep breathing exercises for a few minutes every day. Taking a "cat nap" is recommended, especially in the summer months. Bottom line, as we age, quality sleep is more important for health than eating.

For the best sleep, wear lose fitted clothing and ensure that all lights are turned off. This includes eliminating light from music devices, radios, cell phones, electronics, etc. At a minimum, turn the angle of the device or cell phone away from you or tape up the light source so that it does not shed light on you. The darkness activates the nerve pathways in the brain that releases melatonin, which in turn regulates sleep, eating, reproduction, etc. A drop in body temperature at night also helps a person sleep better. Therefore, do no use an electric blanket unless medically necessary. If needed, use layers of blankets or wear a lose sweater, pants and socks (yes socks if your feet get too cold at night) to bed.

The best posture for sleeping is on your side with the back slightly curled. This is often referred to as the fetal position. If needed, place a pillow between your knees to reduce pressure on the sciatic nerve. The next best posture is sleeping on your back. Place a pillow under your head and, if needed, under your neck to ensure that your back is straight. To target lower back problems, place a pillow under the knees, encouraging a more natural spinal curvature. Most people shift positions during sleep. If possible, try to establish these two positions as much as possible. If you cannot find a quality mattress, an alternative is to place a comforter, a light mattress, or a mattress topper on the floor and sleep there as the flat surface of the floor will help align your body and the mattress overlay will keep the sleeping area soft.

In today's world, there are too many stresses in most peoples' lives so rest and sleep are even more crucial to keep our bodies running smoothly. People who do not sleep enough generally hold onto fat and have a hard time losing weight. Bottom line, you cannot get healthy and lose weight (and keep it off) unless you give your body proper rest on a nightly (or daily if you work a night shift) basis.

A few words regarding the sleep schedule and its impact on health. In the old days, before the days of electricity, people went to bed shortly after dark and then got up in the middle of the night—at which time they prayed, talked or read or wrote by candlelight, etc.—and then went back to sleep. They engaged in what is know as bicameral sleep. A two-part sleep that allowed for sufficient rest as well as time for prayer, contemplation, communication, and creativity. The added benefit of this sleep schedule was that humans had a very regular sleeping schedule; they were connected with (and dependent on) the sun and the moon and thus their hormones were in true balance. Humans are designed to sleep at dusk as the ensuing night approaches and awaken as morning dawn breaks. Thus, try to align your sleep and waking cycle to the sun and the moon as much as possible. If you cannot do so for whatever reason, ensure that you have a regular sleep schedule and that you get sufficient sleep.

Before going to sleep each night, do something for yourself, even if it is just thinking one kind and gentle thought. Things happen to you but they don't make you. You make you. Remember the kind, loyal and gentle person that you are. So, spend a few minutes each day making yourself a loving person, and connecting with and loving yourself.

13 DENTAL HEALTH

If your teeth and gums look healthy, most likely you are also physically healthy. Your health status is generally reflected in your dental health, and vice versa.

Keep a close eye on your dental health. If your gums or teeth hurt, you may be low on Vitamin D or your carbohydrate intake may be too high. It could be some other problem or reason as well. If you have cavities, possibly your diet needs to be adjusted to reduce blood sugar levels. Good dental health is not just about brushing teeth. What you eat and how healthy you are is reflected in your teeth and gums. Certainly, good dental hygiene is important but so is good nutrition. If your nutritional profile seems excellent but your dental health remains weak, do not stop there. Look further into what your body needs. Perhaps you are eating right but your body is not providing proper nutrition to your bones and teeth. Could it be that you have digestive issues or food sensitivities that block nutrients from reaching the parts of your body where they are needed. Do not stop, continue to figure out what is going on with your body.

A few words about the importance of nutrition and

dental health. It is essential that anyone trying to clean up their diet, ensure they are getting proper nutrition. As discussed in Chapter 11, individuals who are vegetarians, vegans, and fruitarians are particularly at risk of not consuming a balanced and nutritious diet. Those eating a plant strong, fiber rich diet can also be at risk. Sometimes those who overeat are able to obtain the full complement of nutrients due to the mere fact of overeating. But, this is not the best way to ensure proper nutrition. As many know, overeating has its own negative health outcomes. (The body reacts to overeating, just the machine that becomes over flooded when too much fuel is injected into it.) Instead, the best way is to periodically track food intake to ensure proper nutritional profile.

The concern regarding nutritional sufficiency of diet applies particularly to children and teenagers who go on such diets without sufficient knowledge about food and nutrition. Their bodies are at a very critical stage of development and proper nutrition is essential for their continued development. It is essential to ensure that they are taking Vitamin B12, Vitamin D, calcium, riboflavin, and protein through food and, if needed, by using supplements. Indeed, done correctly, one can obtain most of their nutritional needs by consuming the right kinds and quantities of whole fruits, vegetables, legumes, grains, and nuts and seeds.

In addition to maintaining proper nutrition, there are various ways in which good dental hygiene can be achieved. For example, an excellent way to clean teeth after every meal is to eat lettuce or some green leafy vegetables at the end of the meal, particularly after eating sugary foods. The lettuce or greens will cleanse the teeth and thus limit the amount of sugar on the teeth. If you have dental issues, at a minimum, rinse your teeth with water after every meal and every snack, and reduce intake of sugary foods (including fruits). In addition to any dental routine, another daily practice may be to use tooth picks to clean out food particles between teeth after each meal. I know someone who uses toothpicks after mealtime. His dentist said that his teeth and gums were in excellent health, which may be due to the fact that he uses toothpicks after every meal. Bottom line, find a way to keep your teeth clean.

For toothpaste, use natural paste that is free of dyes and chemicals. In addition to regular brushing, rinsing the mouth and gargling with salt water every night can be helpful if dealing with a sore throat. Periodically rinse the mouth with a natural antiseptic such as water with a few drops of Tea Tea Oil or Oil of Oregano. These measures are relatively simple and highly cost effective.

14 THE HOME

Having modified your daily diet and exercise regimen, there are additional steps that can be taken to achieve greater health.

Look at the environment where you live, sleep, play and breathe. What is your body being exposed to each day? Do you use shampoos, soaps, and other items etc. Do you know the chemicals found in these products? Many commercial preparations contain unhealthy chemicals. Switch to a milder preparation or make your own home-made preparations if this is an issue. You can also occasionally shower without soap and just use water and a washcloth for scrubbing. For shampoo and conditioner, you can occasionally apply the "no poo" method, which calls for not using a commercial shampoo or conditioner. At times, just using water to rinse out your hair may be sufficient. Baking soda and vinegar can also replace shampoo and conditioner, respectively. Alternatively, milder commercial preparations should be considered. There are many such preparations in the market. In addition, washing hair fewer times per week is actually healthier as this allows the body sufficient time to replenish the scalp and hair with natural oils. The natural oils make hair feel softer, stronger and healthier.

To the extent possible, use natural products on your body. This includes deodorant. Use a natural, non-aluminum deodorant or possibly go without deodorant if the weather permits. Alternatively, a simple deodorant preparation can be made using baking soda, cornstarch, and some essential oil. If needed, coconut oil can be added to the preparation. Lemon juice is another alternative as a deodorant. There are many ways that the use of harsh chemical-laden products can be reduced and preferably avoided.

Carefully review the commercial beauty products that you use, many cosmetics are laced with toxic chemicals. In addition to healthier products in the marketplace, there are home-based substitutes for basic beauty products. Coconut oils works as well or better than most facial creams, lotions, and conditioners. Cornstarch is an alternative for facial or body powder. For eye shadow, blueberry juice is an excellent choice. For blush and lipstick, rubbing the cheeks and lips with a small piece of beet or beet powder works very well. The bottom line is to cut out (or if that is not possible, dramatically reduce) exposure to chemicals that may seep into your body via various pores and orifices. If going to a wedding or some major event, commercial makeup can be used, but use it sparingly.

How about the kitchen? What do you use to wash your dishes. Have you considered the toxic materials in dishwashing detergent or soap. Cleaning dishes is important and sparkling dishes look good, but lacing them with toxic substances is dangerous for health. Use a milder and healthier dish detergent and use ample hot water to ensure the dishes are clean. Also, consider the materials comprising pots and pans and dishes. Teflon is toxic and is not healthy. Dishes embellished with excessive designs or colors are generally laced with toxic chemicals. Simple clear glass dishes may be a better alternative. Invest in high quality products for use in your kitchen. After all, the most important thing is your health and a key determinant of health is what goes inside your body. So, ensure that everything involved in preparing, serving, and consuming food is low toxic or non-toxic.

Ensure that water, particularly drinking water, is high quality and that it is checked annually. If needed, use a high quality water filter for all drinking water. If possible, install a whole house water filter. If concerned about bacteria in the water, boil it prior to use. This approach can also be used for drinking water by cooling down the water after boiling. If highly concerned about water quality, consume organic watery fruits and vegetables (e.g., grapes, oranges, watermelon, tomatoes) instead of water. Bottled water and water-based bottled drinks should also be considered if conditions warrant.

Finally, consider all other chemicals to which you may be exposed. For example, what detergent do you use for washing clothes. What other chemicals are around you? Are your household cleansers such as the countertop and floor cleaning products toxic? How about wall paint and paint thinners. Review the chemicals that you may use on your lawn and yard. Drastically reduce your exposure to these chemicals. One simple alternative to household cleansers is to use vinegar, baking soda and lemon juice for making non-toxic home-made cleansers. It is impossible to completely eliminate exposure to harsh chemicals, but your daily exposure load can be significantly reduced.

15 THE ENVIRONMENT

In the process of aligning your diet toward health, it is important to understand the world around you. One thing that humans often forget is that we are animals—albeit with more advanced brains, a very complex social structure, etc. We are animals and we are connected with nature—we are actually part of nature. Thus, we thrive when we align our lifestyle harmoniously with nature.

We are intimately (and intricately) designed for the planet on which we reside. Our heart, lungs, organs and our entire body are all designed for this planet. In the same way, our brains are designed and wired to help us navigate this planet using our bodies, arms, hands, legs, feet, etc. Our brains and bodies are adapted to the sun, the moon, the air, water, ground, etc. The more that we realize this connection, the greater health we can achieve. This is why we need to eat whole foods and drink plenty of fresh water.

We also need to spend time in nature each day and get our daily dose of fresh air and sunshine. At the end of the day, as dusk approaches, we need to prepare for rest and relaxation and sleep in a blissful slumber. We are part of nature and we need to fill our bodies with the goodness of the planet in order to achieve health. Doing all of these things helps anyone achieve a svelte and healthy body, i.e., one that is full of vitality and energy.

Wholesome and living foods are made by nature and they are designed to be consumed. As mentioned earlier, whole foods are actually bio-compatible with our bodies and organ systems, and particularly needed to nourish our brains and bodies. It may be hard to believe, but fruits and vegetables need to be eaten to propagate themselves. By eating ripe whole fruits we and other animals release the seeds and allow them to spread. We help perpetuate the planet and thus eating whole foods is one of our primal goals to help the planet. Certainly, if consuming something, e.g., peanuts, causes discomfort or perhaps an allergic reaction, then please discontinue its use. Else, eat all the whole foods that are compatible with your body and system.

In addition, connect with the earth every day. No matter what the weather is on a given day, spending at least a few minutes outdoors playing , walking, touching trees and plants or perhaps gardening. Today, humans spend too much time indoors and to much time touching computers, cell phones, TVs, etc. This makes it even more important that we ground our bodies and diffuse any electrical charge. The easiest way to do this is to touch the earth and the trees and plants in nature.

If you feel inclined, to occasionally eat some milk, cheese, yogurt, eggs, meat etc., this is fine. However, in that case, you need to thank the animal that provided these things to you. If possible, you also need to care for the animals who provided you with "food." For example, if a cow or goat provides you milk, ideally you need to give them, in return, food that they would normally eat, shelter to protect them, e.g., from wild animals, floods, thunderstorms. This is how symbiotic relationships work. This used to be the way humans and animals such as goats, sheep, chickens, buffalos, and cows "worked together" with humans. Similarly, cats and dogs used to provide warmth and protection to humans by sleeping at their feet and serving as blankets in return for food and shelter. In modern day life, this is not always possible as many people do not have room to raise cows or goats, but be aware that this is how it should be—there should be give and take rather than just taking. Find your own way to give back to the animals and to the earth. Perhaps by supporting the farmers who raise animals in an ethical manner. At the very least, help protect the environment in which they live. In the process, you will help improve the environment for yourself and everyone else. We should all help protect the environment.

The above notwithstanding, consuming meat, eggs, and dairy should not be a habit. These foods should be consumed sparingly, if at all. We should respect the lives of other creatures and consume them and their milk, eggs etc. only on occasion (e.g., on special holidays) and if necessary. Eating animal-based products is not necessary and research has shown that individuals who obtain their full complement of nutrients through plant sources are much healthier.

Living a life connected with nature will not only help advance your physical health, it will awaken your spirit. It will open your eyes, ears, heart and mind; and it will help you see the world in a totally new light. You will see that you are very intimately interconnected with life on earth and with nature. It will spawn a whole new level of consciousness within you.

There are two things that are important in life—to seek knowledge and love. When you open your eyes to the world and how it works, you will have obtained some knowledge of this world and at the same time achieve a level of understanding (love) of life and all the things that support it.

16 MORAL SUPPORT

Your assumptions are your windows on the world. Scrub them off every once in a while, or the light won't come in."
Isaac Asimov

A change in lifestyle can often be very hard to achieve. But, if gains in health and energy are the rewards, then the seeds for the journey to a new life can be readily sown.

If you need advice on how to move forward, remember that you are what you achieve every day. If excellence in health and well being is what you are striving for, then make the lifestyle change. Once you have adopted new ways of eating, drinking and living, they will become habits if you remember the rewards that the new path provides. It may not seem like it now, but with time (yes time will be required to revert back to health but it will happen) the new lifestyle will eventually become a habit, and a truly rewarding one as well.

As they say, life is not about where you start or where you end up, its the journey that you undertake and the distance that you cover that matters. So, don't say "I am too busy right now" or "I don't have the freedom or the path to this new way of living" This is the time for your path and your journey has already begun. You never know your potential until you chart the waters of the impossible.

Everybody wants things to happen to their interest and desire, but they don't always want to put the work and effort into it or they don't know how to get there. Stop thinking and put the energy into achieving your goals day by day. Do not wait any longer. Stop trying to learn from everybody else, believe in yourself and your ability to transform yourself into something good and possibly something great.

As someone once said "this comfort zone you are currently in is a danger zone." It may seem comfortable in one sense (as it is what you have and are used to), but it may be neither truly comfortable nor safe and it is stopping you from reaching your true potential. You are always a lot more than you realize, and you have more will power and strength inside of you than you think, so stop selling yourself short. You have to rewrite your own (his/ her) story of life, stop listening to everyone who says that this is the way it is, and that you cannot lose weight and get healthier. Learn from those who have succeeded. Failure is part of the path to success. I failed for over 30 years before I succeeded. You fail a thousand times before you succeed, every single person does. It is the losers who fail a few times and quit and stop there. Keep trying and you will most definitely get there. Don't be a quitter.

As someone once said, "The loser and the winner both fail, its just that the winner gets back up again and again." There are no shortcuts in achieving what you want in life. Remember, no pain no gain. If you want to make real progress then you really have to look at your life in a different way, you have to say "I have to take control of this process and not just hope that it's going to work out like people do when they make a resolution on New Year's day." Go out there and start your journey. You can reach your goals or perhaps even go beyond.

If you are struggling, then get in touch with me and I will step in and help.

17. FIGHTING ILLNESSES

If you or someone you know is fighting an illness, in particular a serious illness such as cancer, heart disease etc., it is important to seek expert medical advice as soon as possible. Life is complex and illness is sometimes not easy to fight. Working with a medical professional gives the individual facing the illness the ability to obtain important medical information through laboratory and other medical tests, to obtain prescription medication, if needed, and to connect with experts in the medical field. Please do not shy away from seeking medical advice in time of need.

The above notwithstanding, there are a host of measures one can to either avoid or to fight illness. Among these, the following measures are strongly recommended for everyone:

1. Avoid carcinogens, basically
    *   avoid all animal products and fish; (in particular, animal fat should be avoided at all costs because of its concentration of pesticides and toxic chemicals).
    *   burned food (the burning process generates toxic chemicals);

- eat organic/spray free whenever possible (if concerned about some fruits and vegetables, at a minimum, do not consume the outer covering/peel of such foods).

2. Avoid hormones, this is basically about avoiding animal products (the human body and cancer is very sensitive to things like IGF1 and estrogen in animal foods).

3. Avoid animal bacteria and viruses, again avoid animal products.

4. Eat lots of fiber as it helps feed the body and clean the digestive system (eat fruits and vegetables)

5. Eat ample antioxidants daily (eat fruits and vegetables).

6. Eat a balanced nutrient rich diet (eat whole foods).

7. Help your body maintain its ideal alkaline environment, which has been proven to be hostile to cancer and other maladies (i.e., eat whole foods and, if needed, drink water dissolved in sodium bicarbonates to achieve alkalinity).

8. Minimize cooking of food to reduce intake of harmful chemical compounds that result from cooking. These compounds are known as advanced glycation end products (AGEs). The best way to reduce AGEs is to cook foods with moist heat, using shorter cooking times, lower temperatures and acidic ingredients such as vinegar or lemon juice. Thus, steaming, stewing or boiling food is preferred over grilling, roasting, broiling or frying them.

9. Laugh at life. Cry when you need to. In the end just laugh.

If you are really concerned about avoiding/ fighting cancer there are a number of foods that have been shown to be good against cancer. They are all plant-based of course. They include turmeric, sweet potatoes, cranberries, flax seeds, etc. And there are other important lifestyle factors that need to be incorporated into your life. This includes maintaining a healthy immune system by staying active, avoiding excessive stress and pollution, and making sure you get enough sleep.

In addition to these changes, there are a number of additional lifestyles measures that can be part of the healing process. These include meditation and laughter. Although these two measures seem to be on the opposing sides of the continuum, they are both crucial for fighting illness.

Meditation is not simply relaxing and taking a break or a nap. It is something much more powerful. As declared by the world's best meditators, immense power can be achieved through meditation. Even though that may not be the goal here, the power of meditation in healing the body is amazing. With meditation, one is able to center their body on the current movement and to allow the breath (and thus oxygen) to reach into all the crevices of the of the body. Meditation allows one to not only be introspective and in the moment, it allows the meditator to step away from reality and to temporarily find an inner sanctuary and to live in that peaceful place. There is no need to think in the inner sanctuary, its just important to breathe. Meditation will boost your immune system and allow inner emotions and trauma to release. Meditation should be practiced every day and as often as possible to heal the body and the mind.

The inner peace that results, will provide strength and allow you to respond to the world more meaningfully. It is a form of brain and body training. Meditation can change the structure of the brain. It helps with depression and anxiety, and it can help fight addiction. The goals is to focus on peace and bring it into your body.

Another element of wellness is fun and laughter. This is no laughing matter but do laugh as your health and your survival may depend on it. Fun and laughter are key to fighting illness. It is through laughter that our bodies begin to "smile" on the inside and thus heal. Although we may not realize it, we are meant to be peaceful and happy and when we engage in fun and laughter and spread it to others, our bodies and minds begin to respond with kindness.

The need for laughter is best presented through the story of an individual who was diagnosed with cancer and told to go home and prepare to die within six weeks. He did not know what to do so he picked up some Vitamin C at the drug store and some funny movies at the video store to take home (this was before the days of online streaming movies). He took the vitamin C daily and spent his days watching funny movies and laughing. To everyone's surprise, he never died from the cancer. What happened? It seemed that with the Vitamin C (which is a powerful antioxidant) and the laughter, his cancer went into remission. Although such luck may not come to everyone, this story expresses the value of experiencing fun and laughter and the value of antioxidants in regaining health. Similarly, when a wise person who suffered a fairly serious brain stroke was asked how he had managed to recover so well in the three ensuing years, he responded "a key aspect to my newfound heath is happiness—one has to chose to be happy in life in order to fight the ravages disease." Focus on simple fun and happiness will follow.

There are many ways to have fun. Playing with children can bring happiness and return us to a simpler time in our own lives. Get dirty if that is what it takes to achieve happiness. Happiness can also be induced through music, art, walking, connecting with nature and many other ways. Choose your own pathway to fun and happiness. Even learn to laugh at yourself and at the world around you and your body will respond with kindness and love.

18 MAINTAINING THE NEW LIFESTYLE

Change is hard, particularly dramatic change. But, such change can be achieved if there are sufficient incentives. A new diet and lifestyle such as the one proposed in this book can be best achieved if one understands the logic and the rationale behind the whole foods diet and, over time, experiences sufficient increases in health and energy on the diet. Then it is easier to continue along the new path and to say "no" to the negative food and lifestyle choices.

There are, in addition, strategies for success that can be utilized to help transition to the new to the new lifestyle. These strategies include:

- Always keep healthy food and water available and nearby.
- When going out for errands, activities etc., ensure that your are not hungry prior to heading out.
- Maintain a periodic log (or estimate) of your daily food and water intake
- Distract yourself in order to avoid overeating—if feeling unnecessarily hungry perhaps go for a walk,

read a book, take a shower, or watch a movie.

- If needed, for a short period of time, cheat so that diet does not become too burdensome.
- Do whatever is necessary to be safe, e.g., if on a road trip and feeling tired and hungry, get coffee and food etc. to ensure that you can continue to drive safely.

Understand that health is a lifestyle change to which you must commit with conviction. It is something you must truly covet. In the end, the rewards will be priceless —a new body that feels stronger, younger, more agile, and energetic. The real reward will be true health, which you will not want to give up at any cost.

Once you achieve success on the diet, the challenge shifts to maintaining the diet and keeping your "new" body. Many individuals lose the weight but have a hard time keeping it off. It is as if your brain and body have a "memory" of their body and its shape. There is also the concept of homeostasis, which is the biological function that wants to keep you the same. Your body gets used to your weight and thus seeks sustain itself in that state. Once you lose weight, a new you emerges and your sense of balance or homeostasis needs to be adjusted. New memories of your body and its shape and size need to be ingrained into the brain. Thus, the border and the outline of the body has to be updated in your mind. Along your health journey, the goal is to replace the memory of the "old" you with the "new" you. Build new memories of your body and erase the old ones. This journey may require that you find an old piece of clothing that once fit you and eventually being able to wear it again. If there are no such clothes, then buy one or two pieces of clothing that would fit you at the end of your health journey and use them to gauge your progress.

To maintain your new habits, you have to be determined else the old habits will come back and take over. In the end, if you maintain your conviction, your reward will be true health—a priceless reward more precious than almost anything else in this world.

19 SUCCESS STRATEGIES

As you begin your journey, do not forget the strategies that are required for achieving a healthy and svelte body. Summarized below are some of the key strategies that will lead to a svelte and healthy body.

Key Strategies

Diet
- Eat whole foods as much as possible—vegetables, whole grains, legumes, nuts and seeds, and some fruit. This is the best way to obtain the key macronutrients—carbohydrates, fats and protein. Smoothies can be added to the diet and consumed periodically. Juices on the other hand should be consumed sparingly. If possible, eliminate juices altogether and consume whole foods instead. If taking juice as part of a diet, ensure that it is low in sugar and salt. If not, add leafy greens to the juice.
- Eat some whole foods in raw form each day. Cooked foods should also be consumed.

- Consume high ORAC (Oxygen Radical Absorbance Capacity, which is a measure of food's antioxidant capacity) foods daily,
- If concerned about bacteria, viruses, etc. in raw food, use ample hot water to clean / lightly boil all food before consuming it.
- Never go hungry except when fasting for religious or other reasons such as a cleanse or due to lack of immediate access to healthy food. Eat well and then take a 2 to 3 hour break before eating again.
- Balance sweet and savory foods in your diet. As the body gets older, excess sugar and salt are generally harder to manage, but not if one takes breaks between meals and balances sugar/salt, e.g., a savory salad with pears or strawberries added.
- Eat leafy greens (only the ones that taste good to your palate) every day. This does not mean eat greens you hate; instead, eat lettuce if that is the leafy green that you like or can handle in sizable quantity.
- Treat fruit as nature's desert, i.e., generally no more than two or three desserts per day unless you are very athletic and need the extra carbohydrates and sugar.
- Do not eat processed grains, e.g., white bread, white pasta, or white rice. Instead, eat the whole grain bread, pasta and brown rice.
- Only eat fruits and vegetables that taste good to your palate.
- Eat legumes and good fats every day; in particular, eat foods containing Omega 3 fatty acids, e.g., flaxseeds, walnuts, and chia seeds.
- Periodically take a high quality vitamin and mineral supplement to ensure that your body is not missing key nutrients.
- Determine and maintain the proper ratio of carbohydrates, fats and protein for your body.
- Use a nutritional tracking tool periodically to ensure

that your diet meets daily nutritional requirements and that the ratio of carbohydrates to fats to protein is maintained.

- Don't forget the fiber. A fiber rich diet is crucial for health and wellness. If you eat whole foods you do not need to worry about fiber as whole food is packed with fiber.
- Ensure proper hydration. Water keeps the organs functioning optimally, makes the skin supple, and it aids the digestive process. Drink water and herbal teas. Smoothies are fine but, as mentioned, consumption of juices and other sugary drinks should limited. Consumption of caffeinated tea and coffee should be limited.
- Consume caffeinated drinks sparingly and hydrate with water afterwards.
- Drink juices sparingly. To the extent possible, consume whole foods rather than extracted juices. If drinking juices add leafy greens to the juice to add fiber and add boiled legumes to smoothies to add protein.
- Drink alcohol very sparingly or avoid completely if possible.

Lifestyle

- Get your rest and sleep soundly.
- Relax and engage in deep breathing exercises daily.
- Get fresh air routinely.
- Think of kind and gentle thoughts before going to sleep.
- Keep your body and surroundings free of heavy chemicals.
- Use meditation to calm and cleanse the body.
- Use fun and humor to bring happiness within.

Exercise

- Move regularly to keep the body "river" flowing; it is also important to sweat to relieve stress and get the toxins out. Sweating can be a sign that the body is working to remove toxins.
- Engage in yoga, tai chi or similar stretch exercises daily to maintain flexibility and balance as you age.
- Moderate exercise is required and variety is the spice of exercise life. Try to make exercise fun (e.g., group sports, dancing, and interval exercises are good).
- Walk regularly to keep your body active without stressing your joints.
- Blood flow is critical for good health.
- Do not over-exercise as this will lead to oxidative stress in the body.
- Stay active and have fun.

BIBLIOGRAPHY

Gregor, Michael, M.D.., and Stone, Gene, *How Not to Die*, MacMillan Children's Publishing, 2015.

Glycemic Load, N.D., *In Wikipedia*

National Institute on Aging, *National Institute of Heath*. Paleolithic Era, *N.D., In Wikipedia*

Richman, George and Anish Sheth, MD, *What's Your Poo Telling You?* San Francisco: Chronicle Books, LLC, 2010.

Richman, George and Anish Sheth, MD, *What's My Pee Telling Me?* San Francisco: Chronicle Books, LLC, 2009.

The U.S. Geological Survey's (USGS) Water Science School, "The Water in You," usgs.gov.

APPENDIX

Healthy Diet
(Source: World Health Organization)

Fact sheet N°394
Updated September 2015

Key facts

A healthy diet helps protect against malnutrition in all its
forms, as well as noncommunicable diseases (NCDs),
including diabetes, heart disease, stroke and cancer.

Unhealthy diet and lack of physical activity are leading
global risks to health.

Healthy dietary practices start early in life – breastfeeding
fosters healthy growth and improves cognitive
development, and may have longer-term health benefits,
like reducing the risk of becoming overweight or obese
and developing NCDs later in life.

Energy intake (calories) should be in balance with energy
expenditure. Evidence indicates that total fat should not
exceed 30% of total energy intake to avoid unhealthy
weight gain (1, 2, 3), with a shift in fat consumption away
from saturated fats to unsaturated fats (3), and towards the

elimination of industrial trans fats (4).

Limiting intake of free sugars to less than 10% of total energy intake (2, 5) is part of a healthy diet. A further reduction to less than 5% of total energy intake is suggested for additional health benefits (5).

Keeping salt intake to less than 5 g per day helps prevent hypertension and reduces the risk of heart disease and stroke in the adult population (6).

WHO Member States have agreed to reduce the global population's intake of salt by 30% and halt the rise in diabetes and obesity in adults and adolescents as well as in childhood overweight by 2025 (7, 8, 9).

Overview

Consuming a healthy diet throughout the life course helps prevent malnutrition in all its forms as well as a range of noncommunicable diseases and conditions. But the increased production of processed food, rapid urbanization and changing lifestyles have led to a shift in dietary patterns. People are now consuming more foods high in energy, fats, free sugars or salt/sodium, and many do not eat enough fruit, vegetables and dietary fibre such as whole grains.

The exact make-up of a diversified, balanced and healthy diet will vary depending on individual needs (e.g. age, gender, lifestyle, degree of physical activity), cultural context, locally available foods and dietary customs. But basic principles of what constitute a healthy diet remain the same.
For adults

A healthy diet contains:

Fruits, vegetables, legumes (e.g. lentils, beans), nuts and whole grains (e.g. unprocessed maize, millet, oats, wheat, brown rice).

At least 400 g (5 portions) of fruits and vegetables a day (2). Potatoes, sweet potatoes, cassava and other starchy roots are not classified as fruits or vegetables.

Less than 10% of total energy intake from free sugars (2, 5) which is equivalent to 50 g (or around 12 level teaspoons) for a person of healthy body weight consuming approximately 2000 calories per day, but ideally less than 5% of total energy intake for additional health benefits (5). Most free sugars are added to foods or drinks by the manufacturer, cook or consumer, and can also be found in sugars naturally present in honey, syrups, fruit juices and fruit juice concentrates.

Less than 30% of total energy intake from fats (1, 2, 3). Unsaturated fats (e.g. found in fish, avocado, nuts, sunflower, canola and olive oils) are preferable to saturated fats (e.g. found in fatty meat, butter, palm and coconut oil, cream, cheese, ghee and lard) (3). Industrial trans fats (found in processed food, fast food, snack food, fried food, frozen pizza, pies, cookies, margarines and spreads) are not part of a healthy diet.

Less than 5 g of salt (equivalent to approximately 1 teaspoon) per day (6) and use iodized salt.

For infants and young children

In the first 2 years of a child's life, optimal nutrition fosters healthy growth and improves cognitive development. It also reduces the risk of becoming overweight or obese and developing NCDs later in life.

Advice on a healthy diet for infants and children is similar to that for adults, but the following elements are also important.

Infants should be breastfed exclusively during the first 6 months of life.

Infants should be breastfed continuously until 2 years of age and beyond.

From 6 months of age, breast milk should be complemented with a variety of adequate, safe and nutrient dense complementary foods. Salt and sugars should not be added to complementary foods.

Practical advice on maintaining a healthy diet
Fruits and vegetables

Eating at least 400 g, or 5 portions, of fruits and vegetables per day reduces the risk of NCDs (2), and helps ensure an adequate daily intake of dietary fibre.

In order to improve fruit and vegetable consumption you can:

  always include vegetables in your meals
  eat fresh fruits and raw vegetables as snacks
  eat fresh fruits and vegetables in season
  eat a variety of choices of fruits and vegetables.

Fats

Reducing the amount of total fat intake to less than 30% of total energy intake helps prevent unhealthy weight gain in the adult population (1, 2, 3).

Also, the risk of developing NCDs is lowered by reducing saturated fats to less than 10% of total energy intake, and trans fats to less than 1% of total energy intake, and replacing both with unsaturated fats (2, 3).

Fat intake can be reduced by:

changing how you cook – remove the fatty part of meat; use vegetable oil (not animal oil); and boil, steam or bake rather than fry;
avoiding processed foods containing trans fats; and
limiting the consumption of foods containing high amounts of saturated fats (e.g. cheese, ice cream, fatty meat).

Salt, sodium and potassium

Most people consume too much sodium through salt (corresponding to an average of 9–12 g of salt per day) and not enough potassium. High salt consumption and insufficient potassium intake (less than 3.5 g) contribute to high blood pressure, which in turn increases the risk of heart disease and stroke (6, 10).

1.7 million deaths could be prevented each year if people's salt consumption were reduced to the recommended level of less than 5 g per day (11).

People are often unaware of the amount of salt they consume. In many countries, most salt comes from processed foods (e.g. ready meals; processed meats like bacon, ham and salami; cheese and salty snacks) or from food consumed frequently in large amounts (e.g. bread). Salt is also added to food during cooking (e.g. bouillon, stock cubes, soy sauce and fish sauce) or at the table (e.g. table salt).

You can reduce salt consumption by:

not adding salt, soy sauce or fish sauce during the preparation of food

not having salt on the table
limiting the consumption of salty snacks
choosing products with lower sodium content.

Some food manufacturers are reformulating recipes to reduce the salt content of their products, and it is helpful to check food labels to see how much sodium is in a product before purchasing or consuming it.

Potassium, which can mitigate the negative effects of elevated sodium consumption on blood pressure, can be increased with consumption of fresh fruits and vegetables.
Sugars

The intake of free sugars should be reduced throughout the lifecourse (5). Evidence indicates that in both adults and children, the intake of free sugars should be reduced to less than 10% of total energy intake (2, 5), and that a reduction to less than 5% of total energy intake provides additional health benefits (5). Free sugars are all sugars added to foods or drinks by the manufacturer, cook or consumer, as well as sugars naturally present in honey, syrups, fruit juices and fruit juice concentrates.

Consuming free sugars increases the risk of dental caries (tooth decay). Excess calories from foods and drinks high in free sugars also contribute to unhealthy weight gain, which can lead to overweight and obesity.

Sugars intake can be reduced by:

limiting the consumption of foods and drinks containing high amounts of sugars (e.g. sugar-sweetened beverages, sugary snacks and candies); and
eating fresh fruits and raw vegetables as snacks instead of sugary snacks.

How to promote healthy diets

Diet evolves over time, being influenced by many factors and complex interactions. Income, food prices (which will affect the availability and affordability of healthy foods), individual preferences and beliefs, cultural traditions, as well as geographical, environmental, social and economic factors all interact in a complex manner to shape individual dietary patterns. Therefore, promoting a healthy food environment, including food systems which promote a diversified, balanced and healthy diet, requires involvement across multiple sectors and stakeholders, including government, and the public and private sector.

Governments have a central role in creating a healthy food environment that enables people to adopt and maintain healthy dietary practices.

Effective actions by policy-makers to create a healthy food environment include:

Creating coherence in national policies and investment plans, including trade, food and agricultural policies, to promote a healthy diet and protect public health:

increase incentives for producers and retailers to grow, use and sell fresh fruits and vegetables;

reduce incentives for the food industry to continue or increase production of processed foods with saturated fats and free sugars;

encourage reformulation of food products to reduce the contents of salt, fats (i.e. saturated fats and trans fats) and free sugars;

implement the WHO recommendations on the marketing of foods and non-alcoholic beverages to children;

establish standards to foster healthy dietary practices through ensuring the availability of healthy, safe and affordable food in pre-schools, schools, other public institutions, and in the workplace;

explore regulatory and voluntary instruments, such as marketing and food labelling policies, economic incentives or disincentives (i.e. taxation, subsidies), to promote a healthy diet; and

encourage transnational, national and local food services and catering outlets to improve the nutritional quality of their food, ensure the availability and affordability of healthy choices, and review portion size and price.

Encouraging consumer demand for healthy foods and meals:

promote consumer awareness of a healthy diet,

develop school policies and programmes that encourage children to adopt and maintain a healthy diet;

educate children, adolescents and adults about nutrition and healthy dietary practices;

encourage culinary skills, including in schools;

support point-of-sale information, including through food labelling that ensures accurate, standardized and comprehensible information on nutrient contents in food in line with the Codex Alimentarius Commission guidelines; and

provide nutrition and dietary counselling at primary health care facilities.

Promoting appropriate infant and young child feeding practices:

implement the International Code of Marketing of Breast-milk Substitutes and subsequent relevant World Health Assembly resolutions;

implement policies and practices to promote protection of working mothers; and

promote, protect and support breastfeeding in health services and the community, including through the Baby-friendly Hospital Initiative.

WHO response

The "WHO Global Strategy on Diet, Physical Activity and

Health" (12) was adopted in 2004 by the World Health Assembly (WHA). It called on governments, WHO, international partners, the private sector and civil society to take action at global, regional and local levels to support healthy diets and physical activity.

In 2010, the WHA endorsed a set of recommendations on the marketing of foods and non-alcoholic beverages to children (13). These recommendations guide countries in designing new policies and improving existing ones to reduce the impact on children of the marketing of unhealthy food. WHO is also helping to develop a nutrient profile model that countries can use as a tool to implement the marketing recommendations.

In 2012, the WHA adopted a "Comprehensive Implementation Plan on Maternal, Infant and Young Child Nutrition" and 6 global nutrition targets to be achieved by 2025, including the reduction of stunting, wasting and overweight in children, the improvement of breastfeeding and the reduction of anaemia and low birth weight (7).

In 2013, the WHA agreed to 9 global voluntary targets for the prevention and control of NCDs, which include a halt to the rise in diabetes and obesity and a 30% relative reduction in the intake of salt by 2025. The "Global Action Plan for the Prevention and Control of Noncommunicable Diseases 2013–2020" (8) provides guidance and policy options for Member States, WHO and other UN agencies to achieve the targets.

With many countries now seeing a rapid rise in obesity among infants and children, in May 2014 WHO set up the Commission on Ending Childhood Obesity. The Commission is developing a report specifying which approaches and actions are likely to be most effective in different contexts around the world.

In November 2014, WHO organized, jointly with the Food and Agriculture Organization of the United Nations (FAO), the Second International Conference on Nutrition (ICN2). ICN2 adopted the Rome Declaration on Nutrition (14) and the Framework for Action (15), which recommends a set of policy options and strategies to promote diversified, safe and healthy diets at all stages of life. WHO is helping countries to implement the commitments made at ICN2.

Strategy documents
Global action plan for the prevention and control of NCDs 2013-2020
Comprehensive implementation plan on maternal, infant and young child nutrition

References

Hooper L, Abdelhamid A, Moore HJ, Douthwaite W, Skeaff CM, Summerbell CD. Effect of reducing total fat intake on body weight: systematic review and meta-analysis of randomised controlled trials and cohort studies. BMJ. 2012; 345: e7666.

Diet, nutrition and the prevention of chronic diseases: report of a Joint WHO/FAO Expert Consultation. WHO Technical Report Series, No. 916. Geneva: World Health Organization; 2003.

Fats and fatty acids in human nutrition: report of an expert consultation. FAO Food and Nutrition Paper 91. Rome: Food and Agriculture Organization of the United Nations; 2010.

Nishida C, Uauy R. WHO scientific update on health consequences of trans fatty acids: introduction. Eur J Clin Nutr. 2009; 63 Suppl 2:S1–4.

Guideline: Sugars intake for adults and children. Geneva: World Health Organization; 2015.

Guideline: Sodium intake for adults and children. Geneva: World Health Organization; 2012.

Comprehensive implementation plan on maternal, infant and young child nutrition. Geneva: World Health Organization; 2014.

Global action plan for the prevention and control of NCDs 2013–2020. Geneva: World Health Organization; 2013.

Global status report on noncommunicable diseases 2014. Geneva: World Health Organization; 2014.

Guideline: Potassium intake for adults and children. Geneva: World Health Organization; 2012.

Mozaffarian D, Fahimi S, Singh GM, Micha R, Khatibzadeh S, Engell RE et al. Global sodium consumption and death from cardiovascular causes. N Engl J Med. 2014; 371(7):624-634.

Global strategy on diet, physical activity and health. Geneva: World Health Organization; 2004.

Set of recommendations on the marketing of foods and non-alcoholic beverages to children. Geneva: World Health Organization; 2010.

Rome Declaration on Nutrition. Second International Conference on Nutrition. Rome: FAO/WHO; 2014.

Framework for Action. Second International Conference on Nutrition. Rome: FAO/WHO; 2014.

Understanding high triglycerides.

http://www.reducetriglycerides.com

SHOULD YOU WORRY ABOUT FRUCTOSE?

How to Live a Long Life

Three Parts:Living a Healthy LifestyleEating a Healthy
DietReducing Stress

Do you want to live to be over 100? If so, the best way to
do it is to take care of your physical and psychological
health during the many years along the way. That way, not
only will you be able to maximize your lifespan, but be
healthy enough to enjoy all of it.

Part 1 of 3: Living a Healthy Lifestyle

1 Prepare your body for a long life by exercising.
Exercise benefits both your physical and mental health.
The physical activity strengthens your body, helps you
control your weight, and improves your balance and
coordination. Simultaneously, your body releases
endorphins which will help you relax and feel good.

Try to do both aerobic exercise and strength training.

Aerobic exercise gets your heart rate up and improves
your endurance. Possible activities include jogging, fast
walking, swimming, and many types of sports. Try to do
150 to 75 minutes per week.

Strength training, like weight lifting, will improve your
bone density and build muscle. Try to do it two times per
week.

Ad

2 Be proactive about identifying and treating health
problems. If you skip doctor's appointments, you increase
the chances of not catching a developing health problem
right at the start. This means that it will likely be more
complicated and harder to treat.[1][2]

Have a checkup once a year. If your doctor
recommends other screenings, do them.

If you have a chronic condition, talk to your doctor
about how to manage it to either improve it or prevent it
from getting worse.

Know what health problems may run in your family
and get screened regularly.

3

Don't take unnecessary risks which could cost you your life. Accidents, including during sports or driving, are frequent causes of head trauma and spinal cord injuries.

Drive carefully, wear your seat belt, and obey speed limits.[3]

Use caution when crossing the street as a pedestrian. Look both ways to see if there are any cars around.

Wear appropriate protective and safety gear when playing sports, particularly risky sports like football, horseback riding, rock climbing, bungee jumping, skydiving, skiing, and snowboarding.

4 Avoid toxic substances that may increase your chances of developing health problems. This includes pollutants, pesticides, chemical fumes, and asbestos.

5

Don't drink too much alcohol. If you do drink, daily recommendations are that women should drink no more than one drink per day and men no more than 1 to 2 drinks per day.[4]

Drinking alcohol in low amounts should be ok for your health as long as you are healthy and don't overdo it.

Excessive drinking can make you more likely to get cancers of the digestive tract, heart problems, strokes, high blood pressure, liver disease, and to suffer injuries in accidents.[5]

If you do drink, be careful not to mix alcohol with medicines, including over-the-counter medicines, that may interact.

Don't drink and drive.

6

Don't shorten your lifespan by smoking. Even if you've smoked for many years, quitting will still improve your health and help you live longer. Smoking greatly increases your risks of:[6]

Lung diseases, including cancer

Cancer of the esophagus, larynx, throat, mouth, bladder, pancreas, kidney, and cervix

Heart attacks

Strokes

Diabetes

Eye disorders like cataracts

Respiratory infections

Gum disease

7

Don't risk your psychological and physical health with street drugs. Street drugs are risky for multiple reasons, both the drug itself may harm you and it may be mixed with other harmful substances. The health risks include:[7]

Dehydration

Confusion

Memory loss

Psychosis

Seizures

Coma

Brain damage

Death

Ad

Part 2 of 3: Eating a Healthy Diet

1 Support your body's ability to heal by eating enough protein. Your body uses protein to make new cells. This means that it is important for repairing tissue damage in your body.[8]

Though meat and animal products are common sources of protein, you can also get all of the proteins you need from plant foods.

Proteins are found in meat, milk, fish, eggs, soy, beans, legumes, and nuts.

Adults should eat 2 to 3 servings of high protein foods per day. Childrens' needs will vary according to their ages.

2

Keep your vitality by enjoying a diet with diverse fruits and vegetables. Fruits are foods that grow from the flower of plants while vegetables are foods that come from the stems, flower buds leaves, and roots. Both are excellent sources of the vitamins and minerals your body needs to stay healthy throughout a long life.[9]

Fruits include berries, beans, corn, peas, cucumber, grains, nuts, olives, peppers, pumpkin, squash, sunflower seeds, and tomatoes. Vegetables include celery, lettuce, spinach, cauliflower, broccoli, beets, carrots, and potatoes.

Fruits and vegetables are low in calories and fat, but high in fiber and vitamins. Eating a diet that is high in fruits and vegetables can reduce your risks of developing cancer, heart problems, high blood pressure, strokes, and diabetes.

Try to eat 4 servings of fruits and 5 servings of vegetables per day.

3

Energize your body for a long life by eating healthy amounts of carbohydrates. Carbohydrates include sugars, starches, and fiber. Your body obtains energy by breaking down these compounds. Simple sugars are digested more quickly than complex sugars.[10]

Simple sugars are found in fruits, milk, milk products, vegetables, and processed sweets.

Complex carbohydrates are in beans, peas, lentils, peanuts, potatoes, corn, green peas, parsnips, whole-grain breads.

About half of your daily calories should come from carbohydrates, with most of it coming from complex carbohydrates as opposed to simple sugars.

4

Eat a limited amount of fat. Your body needs some fat to help it absorb fat soluble vitamins, control inflammation, clot blood and maintain proper brain function, but too much is not good.[11]

Common sources of fats are butter, cheese, whole milk, cream, meats, and vegetable oils.

Eating too much fat increases your chances of high cholesterol, heart problems, and strokes. You can reduce your fat consumption by eating lean meats, poultry, fish, and drinking low-fat milk.[12]

Many restaurants enhance the flavor of their foods with ingredients that are high in fat such as cream, whole milk, or butter. By cooking your food yourself, you can control the amount of fat in your food.

5

Get enough vitamins and minerals through a healthy diet. If you are eating a balanced diet, you are probably getting sufficient vitamins and minerals. These substances are vital for your body to function properly, repair itself and grow.[13]

Vitamins and minerals occur naturally in many foods, especially fruits, vegetables, whole grains, meats, and dairy.

If you are concerned that you may not be getting enough vitamins and minerals, talk to your doctor about adding some multivitamin and multi-mineral supplements to your diet.

The needs of pregnant women and children may differ from the needs of others.

6

Eat a low salt diet. While your body needs some salt too so that you maintain muscle and nerve function and manage your blood volume and pressure and blood volume, too much over a long period of time is unhealthy. [14]

Too much salt can cause high blood pressure and aggravate heart, liver, or kidney conditions.

Most foods contain some salt naturally and many have salt added to enhance the flavor.

Adults should consume no more than about a teaspoon of salt per day. If you have a health condition, you may need to eat much less.

Avoid fast food. Not only is it high in fat, but it is also usually very high in salt.

7

Cleanse your body by drinking enough water. Drinking enough water will help your body flush out toxins, maintain your bodily functions, and keep your kidneys healthy.[15]

Adults may need up to 4 liters of water per day. The amount you need will be influenced by your body weight, your activity level, and the climate you live in.

The best way to stay hydrated is to drink enough water that you don't feel thirsty.

If you urinate infrequently or pass dark or cloudy urine, you probably need to drink more.

ABOUT THE AUTHOR

The author of this book took too long to regain her health, but she ultimately figured it out. Now she feels compelled to share her findings with everyone. She says "I feel for anyone who is suffering from ill health or is overweight. I am here to share my story and hope that it will help others in someway." Once she figured out what is required to achieve good health, she lost 50 pounds and got rid of her pre-diabetic condition and fatty liver disease. She also fought her way back from a nearly collapsed lung. Today, she rarely struggles with asthma, which used to be a debilitating illness for her. She can be reached at sachsweb@gmail.com.